Rheumatology for General Practitioners

Oxford General Practice Series 11

H. L. F. CURREY
Professor of Rheumatology,
London Hospital Medical College

SALLY HULL
Lecturer in General Practice,
The London Hospital and St Bartholomew's Hospital
General Practitioner,
Stepney, London

OXFORD   NEW YORK   TOKYO
OXFORD UNIVERSITY PRESS

Oxford University Press, Walton Street, Oxford OX2 6DP
Oxford New York
Athens Auckland Bangkok Bombay
Calcutta Cape Town Dar es Salaam Delhi
Florence Hong Kong Istanbul Karachi
Kuala Lumpur Madras Madrid Melbourne
Mexico City Nairobi Paris Singapore
Taipei Tokyo Toronto
and associated companies in
Berlin Ibadan

Oxford is a trade mark of Oxford University Press

Published in the United States by
Oxford University Press Inc., New York

British Library Cataloguing in Publication Data
Currey, H. L. F.
Rheumatology for General Practitioners.—(Oxford general practice
series; 11).
1. Arthritis—Treatment. 2. Rheumatism—Treatment
I. Title II. Hull, Sally
616.7'206 RC933
ISBN 0-19-261657-9

Library of Congress Cataloging in Publication Data
Currey, H. L. F. (Harry Lloyd Fairbridge)
Rheumatology for General Practitioners.
(Oxford general practice series; 11)
(Oxford medical publications)
Bibliography: p.
Includes index.
1. Rheumatism. 2. Arthritis. I. Hull, Sally.
II. Title. III. Series: Oxford general practice series;
no. 11. IV. Series: Oxford medical publications.
[DNLM: 1. Joint Diseases. W1 OX55 no. 11/WE 300 C976r]
RC927.C865 1987D 616.7'23 87-7654
ISBN 0-19-261657-9 (pbk.)

Printed and bound in Great Britain by
Biddles Ltd, Guildford and King's Lynn

OXFORD MEDICAL PUBLICATIONS

Rheumatology for General Practitioners

OXFORD GENERAL PRACTICE SERIES

1. Paediatric problems in general practice
   M. Modell and R. H. Boyd
2. Geriatric problems in general practice
   G. Wilcock, J. A. M. Gray, and P. M. M. Pritchard
3. Preventive medicine in general practice
   edited by J. A. M. Gray and G. H. Fowler
5. Locomotor disability in general practice
   edited by M. I. V. Jayson and R. Million
6. The consultation: an approach to learning and teaching
   D. Pendleton, P. Tate, P. Havelock, and T. P. C. Schofield
7. Continuing care: the management of chronic disease
   edited by J. C. Hasler and T. P. C. Schofield
8. Management in general practice
   P. M. M. Pritchard, K. B. Low, and M. Whalen
9. Modern obstetrics in general practice
   edited by G. N. Marsh
10. Terminal care at home
    edited by R. Spilling
11. Rheumatology for GPs
    H. L. F. Currey and S. A. Hull
12. Women's problems in general practice
    edited by A. McPherson

Preface

Rheumatological complaints, whether of the joints or soft tissue, represent a large part of the typical general practitioner's work. Many of these complaints occur amongst the elderly, and the proportion will therefore rise as the number of elderly in the population increases. The investigation and treatment of common rheumatological problems can be supervised by the interested general practitioner in the surgery. It is the authors' belief that primary care is the appropriate place for the management of these conditions, leaving the specialist services to their proper functions; namely advice and consultation, when the general practitioner is in doubt, and the investigation and review of unusual conditions. Well organized 'shared-care' schemes for chronic rheumatic conditions would also enable more general practitioners to participate usefully in the management of chronic conditions.

This book is for the general practitioner who wants to extend his knowledge and practical application of rheumatology, so that he may take a more central role in the management of his patients. With this in mind it provides: a succinct, systematic account of modern rheumatology; a practical guide to the management of the common rheumatological disorders, including instructions on techniques such as how to give local injections, the use of drugs, physiotherapy, and simple appliances as well as the role of manipulative medicine and other alternative therapies; and a guide to the management of the major rheumatic disorders (such as rheumatoid arthritis) which may require collaboration between general practice, rheumatologist, and paramedical services.

The first eight chapters cover the major rheumatological conditions and can be read as a systematic account of current thinking in rheumatology. The later chapters are arranged by region of the body, and offer a more problem-oriented approach to the common conditions met in practice. The emphasis is on conditions met frequently: rare conditions are mentioned briefly, but cannot be covered comprehensively in a book of this size. Key references for a fuller account of specific topics are listed at the end of each chapter.

We have been helped by a number of colleagues who have read and criticized the text. In particular we would like to acknowledge our debts to Dr Dene Egglestone, Dr Christopher Kennard, and Dr Robert Senior.

London   H.L.F.C.
August 1986   S.A.H.

v

Contents

1 Rheumatology and primary care

WHAT IS RHEUMATOLOGY?

Rheumatology is a young speciality with diverse origins. Until recently many units were called departments of physical medicine, reflecting a past association with physical methods of treatment and rehabilitation rather than with specific diagnostic categories. At present there is considerable overlap with other specialities, in particular immunology, neurology, orthopaedics, and metabolic medicine. It is difficult to get a generally agreed definition of a discipline which is still evolving rapidly, but a good working definition is, 'that branch of medicine which deals with the diagnosis and management of disorders of the joints and connective tissue'.

A specialist in rheumatology needs to be a general physician, a specialist in the management of joints and connective tissue, a competent immunologist, and a knowledgeable orthopaedic physician. He must also be able to give sound advice on the rehabilitation of patients with rheumatic disability.

As the speciality is relatively new, many general practitioners feel they have not had adequate training early in their careers to equip them to manage the kind of problems met with in practice. This is not an insurmountable problem. As clinicians we are continually having to cope with new treatments, and occasionally with new disease concepts. The philosophy running throughout this book is that the majority of patients with rheumatic disorders are best managed in the context of primary medical care with occasional forays to the hospital for specialist investigation and review.

THE RANGE OF RHEUMATOLOGY IN GENERAL PRACTICE

It is common experience that rheumatic problems and minor trauma form a considerable bulk of a GP's workload. The most comprehensive analysis of diagnostic categories and consultation rates in general practice comes from the second National Morbidity Survey (OPCS 1979). This survey looked at a selected group of practices over a twelve-month period. Although there is tremendous variation between practices according to such factors as location, age structure, rate of referral to hospital, and the doctor's particular interests, the figures give some idea of the rate at which rheumatological conditions are seen in practice (Tables 1.1 and 1.2).

Table 1.1. *The annual consultation rate per thousand population for a number of chronic conditions compared with the number of individuals attending with that diagnosis per thousand population. This gives an indication of the pattern of follow up for chronic illness in general practice.* (OPCS 1979).

Condition	Consultation rate per 1000 population	Patients consulting per 1000 population
Diabetes	19.3	4.7
Anxiety neurosis	79.4	36.2
Depression	107.6	36.2
Epilepsy	9.1	3.0
Hypertension	90.7	19.9
Congestive heart failure	24.5	5.9
Chronic bronchitis	33.8	10.2
Asthma	31.9	9.6
Osteoarthritis and allied conditions	42.7	17.3
Rheumatoid arthritis and allied conditions	16.8	4.5

Table 1.2. *Breakdown of the range of rheumatic diseases seen in general practice. Taken from the OPCS survey (1979), it shows the annual consulting rates for various rheumatic conditions.*

Condition	Consultation rate per 1000 population
Back disorders	
Spondylosis (including cervical spine)	15.5
Lumbago	12.2
Displaced intervertebral disc	19.1
Back pain alone	21.6
Back pain with sciatica	9.4
Other rheumatic disorders	
Osteoarthritis and allied conditions	42.7
Rheumatoid arthritis	16.8
Non-articular rheumatism	21.6
Frozen shoulder	3.3
Knee disorders	5.7
Gout	4.3

ORGANIZATION OF CARE IN CHRONIC DISEASE

Educational needs

Medical education enables students and young doctors to learn about the diagnosis and treatment of acute episodes of illness. As most junior posts only last a few months, however, it is more difficult to learn about the long-term management of chronic disease by experience. Thus, the doctor entering general practice may not have had an adequate opportunity to acquire the skills needed to organize and carry out the care of a patient with a chronic disease which does not have a cure. The overall objectives for managing patients with chronic disease fall into three categories:

1. Management of the organization of care.
2. Management of the doctor–patient relationship, and effective use of the consultation.
3. Management of the disease process. This will be covered in subsequent chapters.

ORGANIZATION OF CARE

Medical records

Medical records perform a number of related functions. They contain an aide memoir of the current state of the illness and its management. In addition they should hold a data base of relevant personal details about the patient, details of preventive procedures undertaken, and a summary of the past medical history. To these basic functions one can add flow sheets for the management of chronic disease. If these are designed carefully they have a number of advantages. First, they can act as a prompt for the doctor to collect specific information, or carry out a specific examination; for example the commonly used 'gold card' prompts the doctor to check the urine, skin, and blood count. Second, they can highlight gradually changing trends in the condition of a patient. For example, the blood pressure of a patient on steroids may be measured regularly at a clinic, but unless the results are charted a gradual but significant change can easily be missed. Third, they can be used to set targets. For example, the acceptable range of blood pressure or blood sugar readings can be built into the design of the card. Examples of simple flow sheets for their chronic rheumatic conditions to be used with the standard Lloyd George envelopes are shown in Figures 1.1 and 1.2. Further ideas on structuring medical records can be found in Zander *et al.* (1978).

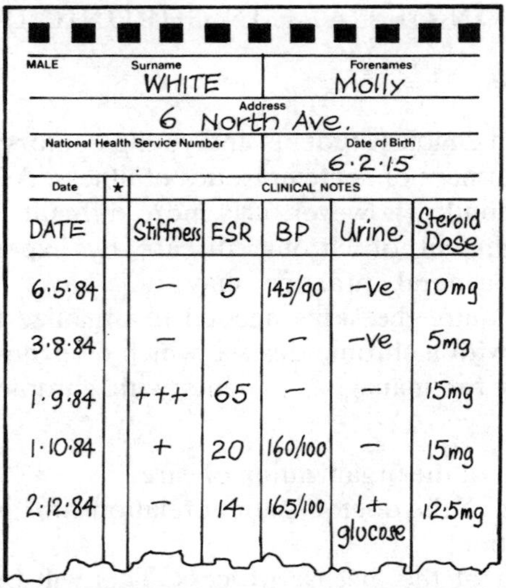

MALE | Surname: WHITE | Forenames: Molly

Address: 6 North Ave.

National Health Service Number | Date of Birth: 6.2.15

Date	★	CLINICAL NOTES				
DATE		Stiffness	ESR	BP	Urine	Steroid Dose
6.5.84		–	5	145/90	–ve	10mg
3.8.84		–		–	–ve	5mg
1.9.84		+++	65	–	–	15mg
1.10.84		+	20	160/100	–	15mg
2.12.84		–	14	165/100	1+ glucose	12.5mg

Fig. 1.1. A simple flow sheet for monitoring key points in a patient with polymyalgia rheumatica on regular steroids.

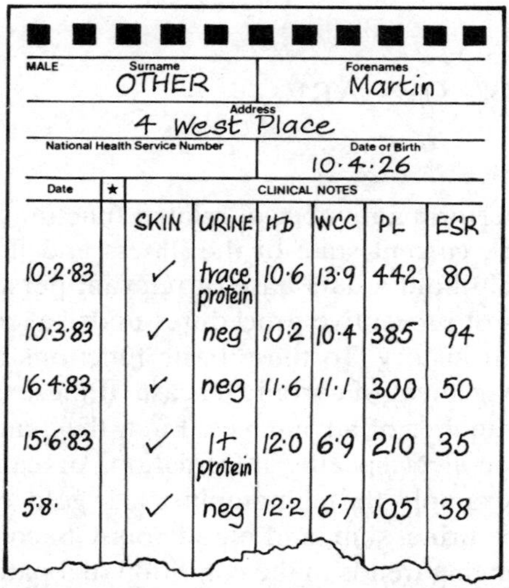

MALE | Surname: OTHER | Forenames: Martin

Address: 4 West Place

National Health Service Number | Date of Birth: 10.4.26

Date	★	CLINICAL NOTES					
		SKIN	URINE	Hb	WCC	PL	ESR
10.2.83		✓	trace protein	10.6	13.9	442	80
10.3.83		✓	neg	10.2	10.4	385	94
16.4.83		✓	neg	11.6	11.1	300	50
15.6.83		✓	1+ protein	12.0	6.9	210	35
5.8.		✓	neg	12.2	6.7	105	38

Fig. 1.2. A cumulative results chart for monitoring patients on slow-acting drugs, such as gold and penicillamine, makes it easy to spot a fall in the platelet count which might otherwise be obscured by improvement in the other indices.

Repeat prescribing

Many patients who have chronic conditions are on regular medication. When organizing a repeat prescription system within a practice it is important to incorporate the following:

1. Built-in arrangements for recalling patients after a limited number of repeat prescriptions. The system must be understood by both staff and patients.
2. A clear indication in patients' notes of their regular medication, how much is to be prescribed, and when the last supply was obtained.

A wide variety of effective repeat-prescription systems are in operation. Some advocate a card held by the patient, others a prescription card in the notes which can be used to audit repeat prescribing and monitor compliance. Whatever system is used it will be seen to be effective if it prevents repeat prescribing with no patient review, alerts the doctor to particular combinations of drugs (e.g. non-steroidal anti-inflammatory drugs and antacids), and registers the cessation of a regular medication. Bolden (1980) gives further suggestions on designing a repeat-prescription system.

Continuity of care

Continuous care by one doctor should help to ensure that observations made about the disease are consistent, and that the management plan is implemented. At the interpersonal level it allows doctor and patient to build up a 'bank' of shared information and trust about one another. This trust becomes important when the disease progresses or problems occur. A good example from another area of general practice is the preliminary work needed to establish the background of trust which enables a terminally ill patient to be managed at home. Many of the vicissitudes of a patient with a chronic condition may call for a similar investment in the doctor–patient relationship. Continuity affects not only consumer satisfaction, but also the outcome of the consultation. For example, it has been shown that compliance with medication is higher when patients consider that they know the doctor well (Ettlinger and Freeman 1981). Unfortunately, both within outpatient departments and within some large group practices, there is an increasing tendency not to see the same doctor at each consultation. There are many defensible reasons for this— holidays, other commitments, trainees, etc—but it can lead to an inappropriate fragmentation of care, either within a group practice or between a number of specialist departments.

The problems which can beset a patient with fragmented care are best illustrated by a case history:

Rose is an overweight 64-year-old housewife with quite severe osteoarthritis affecting her right hip and both knees. She is unable to manage the stairs in her block of flats and is hardly getting out, which makes her depressed. Her GP has tried her on a range of non-steroidal anti-inflammatory drugs, which give her moderate pain relief, and referred her for physiotherapy, but she was unable to get there. She tearfully asks what else can be done, and is referred to the local rheumatologist for supervision. The registrar sees her in the clinic, refers her to the psychiatrist for her depression and requests an orthopaedic opinion on her hip. The surgeon does not think that her hip merits surgery but thinks her moderate hypertension should be supervised in medical outpatients. She fails to attend subsequent appointments saying she has to wait so long in clinic and the ambulance arrives at 8.30 am—if it arrives at all. She becomes more fed up, and sees her GP again some months later, saying, 'If the hospital can't help me I suppose no one can. I'll just have to live with it', and settles into a phase of dissatisfied invalidity.

All doctors will recognize this sequence of events. Sometimes they appear to be inevitable, but they are due to inadequate thought about management objectives and no proper contract being made with the patient about what is treatable and who is most appropriate to treat it. In this case the multiple referrals may have been viewed by the patient as a rejection, both of herself and of her apparently complex and insoluble problems. Certainly a fresh start at sorting out her problems will be more difficult with the anxieties created by previous attempts. This case illustrates a further problem with fragmented care, which Balint (1957) called 'the collusion of anonymity', a state in which no one takes overall direction of the patient's diseases and there is a failure to understand them in the context of the patient's life.

If continuity of care benefits both patients and doctors, then it should become an important objective of practice organization. Its achievement should be regularly reviewed and not be left to chance or to the long-standing traditions of the practice.

THE GENERAL PRACTICE CONSULTATION

Much research has been devoted to the consultation in general practice. It is now established that certain communication skills can be learned, and that the doctor's performance in the consultation can be altered. In turn, it has been shown that altering the performance of the doctor can affect such things as patient satisfaction with medical care, compliance with treatment and understanding of the patient's medical condition.

Many aspects of this subject are relevant to the satisfactory delivery of care to patients with chronic disease. Only two will be discussed here; a good review of the subject can be found in Pendleton and Hasler (1983) *Doctor–patient communication.*

Patients' health beliefs

It is well established that up to half of medical advice is not acted upon. This is often attributed to the giving of inadequate or inappropriate information to the patient. The assumption behind this idea is that there is an automatic progression from the receipt of more information to a change in attitude, resulting in altered behaviour.

Although doctors frequently fail to give adequate information, there is, in addition, a gap between knowledge and action which is well recognized by every physician.

Millie is a 60-year-old spinster with rheumatoid arthritis that has affected her wrists, knees and shoulders for the past six years. She has tried almost every brand of non-steroidal anti-inflammatory drug. Most caused her indigestion, and the others made her worse. For a while she did quite well on regular gold injections, but over a period of eighteen months the disease escaped control. For a period she just took paracetamol saying that she didn't want to take tablets which may cause side-effects, but as the condition got worse she was persuaded to try penicillamine. This did not appear to be helping at all, and on looking at her repeat prescription requests it became clear that her compliance was irregular, although this was denied on confrontation. She then reported that they made her sick, and she would rather have paracodol. She continued to complain bitterly about the pain and stiffness, which exasperated her GP. Eventually she began to see another partner, who felt equally unable to help her.

Here is a patient who has a serious physical condition which can probably be improved by appropriate treatment, yet she persistently fails to engage in treatment and at times seems to sabotage it. Recent studies which have examined the ideas patients have about the nature of disease and medical intervention, have demonstrated the importance of exploring and changing these if a useful working contract is to be achieved by doctor and patient. Health beliefs are as important as medical information in determining behaviour.

The best validated health belief model is that of Becker (1974) which includes the following components:

1. Health motivation—The person's degree of interest in health matters.
2. Susceptibility and severity—The perceived degree of vulnerability to the disease, and the effects it would have on the person's life.
3. Benefits and costs—The perceived benefits of action weighed against the financial cost, or the cost of personal change.
4. Cues to action—These may be internal, e.g. symptoms, or external such as pressure from family or work.

Health beliefs are a combination of information, firmly held traditions and emotional attitudes. It is possible to alter them, but only when they have been made explicit during the course of a consultation. Examining videotaped consultations has shown that the most frequently ignored part of the consultation is exploring the health beliefs of patients and finding out their expectations of medical treatment. This may go some way to explain the extent of failure of compliance.

USES OF THE DOCTOR–PATIENT RELATIONSHIP

The doctor–patient relationship in general practice was first seen as an appropriate subject for study by Michael Balint. The ideas generated from his seminars and books have provided a cohesive ideology for general practice, as well as stimulating the development of techniques for using the doctor–patient relationship in diagnosis and treatment.

Diagnosis

Many patients attend their doctors to get a sympathetic hearing of their problems. Sometimes listening alone is sufficient both to make a diagnosis and a major part of treatment. On other occasions a sympathetic understanding of the patient's emotions can be an important tool in clarifying the problem.

Mrs Jones was 57 years old and had mild osteoarthritis of the hands and knees. She had attended the surgery on two occasions concerned about the development of Heberden's nodes, saying that she supposed she would have to give up her knitting now. She did not seem reassured by the doctor's explanation and continued to attend frequently with aches and pains. Some months later, when she attended again for her hands, the doctor commiserated with her by saying, 'It must be worrying to have pains in your hands which won't go away'. This expression of sympathy enabled her to tell him about her mother who had severe arthritis and needed her constant attention before she died, and from there the doctor could begin to deal with the real fears she had about her illness.

The doctor–patient relationship provides the emotional environment of the consultation. It is the background against which effective communication can take place, but effective use of the relationship also requires the doctor to become aware of his own emotional responses, and how he is being used by the patient at a particular time. This understanding can, on occasion, be of value in clarifying the problems a patient brings to the doctor.

Treatment

Balint (1957) first explored the concept of the doctor as a drug, and demonstrated that advice and reassurance were the two commonest forms in which the 'drug doctor' was administered. Listening and sympathetic understanding have already been mentioned as forms of treatment; their value to the patient is often underrated. On other occasions the doctor may need to use the authority invested in his role, for example to enable a patient with a chronic illness to relinquish certain responsibilities, or to trust in an unknown drug or investigation. Not infrequently the doctor may need to take on a counselling role. For this he must relinquish much of his authority, diminish his social distance from the patient, and move towards a more intimate relationship so that they may examine a problem together.

CONCLUSION

This chapter has attempted to outline the range and frequency of rheumatological complaints in general practice. The importance of good practice organization has been stressed because it forms an essential background for the care of patients with chronic disease. Of equal importance is the ability to communicate effectively with patients. This is particularly significant in chronic conditions where doctor and patient may need to sustain a working relationship over many years.

REFERENCES

Balint, M. (1957). *The doctor, his patient and the illness.* Tavistock, London.

Becker, M. H. (1974). The health belief model and personal illness behaviour. *Hlth Educ. Monogr.* **2**, 328–35.

Bolden, K. J. (1980). Repeat prescription system. *J. R. Coll. Gen. Pract.* **30**, 378.

Ettlinger, P. and Freeman, G. (1981). General practice compliance study: Is it worth being a personal doctor? *Br. med. J.* **282**, 1192–4.

Office of Population Censuses and Surveys (1979). *Morobidity statistics from general practice: Second national study 1971–1972.* HMSO, London.

Periera Gray, D. (1979). The key to personal care. *J. R. Coll. Gen. Pract.* **29**, 666–78.

Pendleton, D. and Hasler, J. (eds) (1983). *Doctor–patient communication.* Academic Press, London.

Zander, L., Beresford, S., and Thomas, P. (1978). Medical records in general practice. Occasional Paper **5** *J. R. Coll. Gen. Pract.*

2 Degenerative joint disease

In common with other body structures, the bones and joints of the skeleton develop changes related to ageing. In the joints this is called *osteoarthritis*, in the bones, *osteoporosis*. Predictably in an ageing population, complaints caused by these conditions increasingly bring patients to the doctor.

The terms used to describe degenerative arthritis are confusing. *Degenerative joint disease* is the general term for all such changes. *Osteoarthritis* and *osteoarthrosis* have the same meaning (degenerative arthritis in a joint which has a synovial cavity), while *spondylosis* refers to degenerative changes in the cartilagenous intervertebral articulations. *Spondylitis*, by contrast, implies inflammatory spinal arthritis, as in ankylosing spondylitis.

OSTEOARTHRITIS	Alternative terms for degenerative changes in	
OSTEOARTHROSIS	synovial joints	Degenerative joint disease
SPONDYLOSIS	Degenerative changes in cartilagenous intervertebral joints	
SPONDYLITIS	Inflammatory arthritis affecting the spine	

EPIDEMIOLOGY

Radiological signs of minor degenerative changes appear in everyone from about the age of 40 years. In most these are associated with minor twinges of pain and stiffness. However, in a minority the process becomes progressive and may lead eventually to joint destruction. While the latter is clearly pathological, some argue that the minor changes, which do not progress, should be regarded as normal age-related events. Degenerative joint disease sufficiently troublesome to make patients consult their GPs is extremely common; thus osteoarthritis of knees, hips and hands, and cervical and lumbar spondylosis account for a significant proportion of a GP's workload (OPCS, 1979). For each consultation relating to rheumatoid arthritis, GPs have about four relating to osteoarthritis and nine relating to problems of backache, spondylosis, disc lesions and sciatica.

Osteoarthritis is referred to as *primary* when no predisposing cause is apparent; the most familiar pattern being that which involves the terminal interphalangeal joints of the fingers to give Heberden's nodes as well as affecting the thumb carpometacarpal joint. This type of osteoarthritis runs in families as an autosomal dominant trait (with incomplete penetrance and expression mainly in females). In osteoarthritis of other joints genetic influences are less obvious.

Secondary osteoarthritis is the term used to describe the degenerative changes which follow abnormal wear in a joint. Most commonly this results from malalignment or irregularity of articular surfaces following trauma, surgery, congenital abnormalities, or abnormal use (Table 2.1). Some argue that all osteoarthritis is secondary in the sense that some minor alteration in joint geometry may have predisposed to it. Normal occupational activities do not predispose to osteoarthritis, and a sedentary life does not protect against it. Vigorous exercise in itself does not necessarily lead to late damage, but some sporting activities may lead to secondary arthritis: wicket-keeper's (or baseball-catcher's) hands and the knees of football players who have suffered recurrent meniscal damage are well known examples.

Table 2.1. *Some causes of secondary osteoarthritis*

Cause	Mechanism
Fractures (shaft)	Malalignment → altered line of weight-bearing
Fractures (through joint)	Irregular bearing surface → scraping abrasion
Skeletal abnormalities: coxa vara; short/long leg	Altered weight-bearing geometry
Other joint diseases: rheumatoid arthitis, osteoarthritis, gout, infections, aseptic necrosis, Perthe's, Paget's	Roughened, irregular bearing surfaces
Internal joint derangements: torn menisci, loose bodies	Abrasion
Hypermobility: torn ligaments, Marfan's syndrome	Instability
Occupational/recreational trauma: ballet-dancers' feet, wicket-keepers' fingers	Recurrent traumatic synovitis
Sensory loss: Charcot's (neuropathic) arthropathy	Loss of protective mechanisms

PATHOGENESIS

Biological joints achieve an efficiency and durability which is well beyond anything possible with man-made articulations. When they do fail through osteoarthritis the important changes start in the hyaline articular cartilage. Two to three millimetres of this tough, resilient material cap the bone ends to provide both a shock-absorbing cushion and a load-bearing surface with extremely low frictional resistance.

It is uncertain whether the initial event is loss of the proteoglycan matrix or fracture of the collagen framework. The first visible change is roughening (fibrillation) of the cartilage surface. Later cartilage loss (ulceration) deepens until eventually raw bone ends become exposed. Attempts at repair are generally ineffective, resulting only in some overgrowth of fibrocartilage. It is not clear why, in most joints, the early changes are not progressive, while in others accelerated wear leads to gross destructive changes. From an early stage bone changes are prominent, with *sclerosis* of the bone ends, outgrowths of new bone (*osteophytes*), and the formation of peri-articular *bone cysts* (containing connective tissue).

The process is more inflammatory than implied by the term degenerative joint disease, and there is evidence that more than just passive wear is involved. Some inflammatory features would be expected to result from the process of clearing wear detritus from the joint surface, but there is speculation that hydroxyapatite crystals (the mineral of bone) may sometimes produce episodes of crystal synovitis (see Chapter 5). Also, the fact that cartilage wear occurs at points not subjected to mechanical stress suggests that other influences may operate. Thus there are suggestions that active enzymatic degradation of matrix by chondrocytes occurs.

CLINICAL FEATURES

As with other types of joint disease the main features of osteoarthritis are pain, stiffness, swelling and loss of function. Pain is not an early feature, probably because articular cartilage is completely insensitive. Indeed, by the time pain appears there are usually some bone changes to be seen on X-ray (unlike the situation in early rheumatoid arthritis). Initially the pain is mild, provoked by activity, and relieved by rest. Later this background of mild pain is punctuated by more acute episodes lasting a few days or longer. During such episodes it may be possible to identify localized, tender, trigger points beside the joint. These may represent sites of peri-articular soft tissue 'strains' which can be treated by a local injection of corticosteroid. Another cause of 'flares' is crystal synovitis caused by the presence of pyrophosphate or hydroxyapatite. With progressive joint destruction the pain becomes more severe, continuous and, in the case of the shoulder, knee or hip, prevents sleep at night. The serious problems of osteoarthritis result mainly from the involvement of weight-bearing joints, particularly the hip and knee, occasionally the ankle, shoulder or elbow.

Stiffness is common, but much less prominent than in rheumatoid arthritis. Characteristically the affected joints gel during a period of inactivity (such as sitting), and it takes a minute or two to loosen up and get going. This is quite different from the prolonged and distressing early morning stiffness of rheumatoid arthritis or polymyalgia rheumatica.

Swelling of an osteoarthritic joint usually occurs as the result of a combination of synovial effusion and bony thickening by osteophytes. The latter is diagnostic of degenerative joint disease, and contrasts with the synovial membrane thickening of rheumatoid arthritis. The other characteristic sign on palpation is coarse crepitus, caused by the movement of raw bone ends against one another. This imparts a grinding sensation to the palpating hand during passive joint movement. The skin overlying an osteoarthritic knee may be warm, but should not be red.

The pattern of joint involvement in primary osteoarthritis is shown in Figure 2.1. The first metatarsophalangeal joint is subject to great mechanical pressures and strains. This may account for its frequent involvement in both osteoarthritis and in gout (Chapter 5).

LABORATORY INVESTIGATIONS

Osteoarthritis is a local condition, thus the erythrocyte sedimentation rate (ESR), haemoglobin and other blood tests should be normal. The synovial fluid is non-inflammatory (protein less than 30 g/l, little or no clot, leucocytes less than 1×10^9/l, neutrophils less than 50 per cent), but there are wide variations.

X-rays are valuable both in establishing the diagnosis and in assessing the severity. Figure 2.2 illustrates the characteristic changes. The diagnostic features are the presence of osteophytes, bone cysts, and bone sclerosis. The severity of damage is indicated by the loss of joint space (indicating cartilage wear).

PARTICULAR PROBLEMS IN OSTEOARTHRITIS

The hip

Before the development of total joint replacement, hip joint involvement was the most important cause of disability in osteoarthritis. The pain may be poorly localized, sometimes being felt exclusively in the knee on that

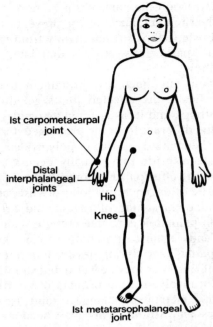

Fig. 2.1. The joints most commonly involved in primary osteoarthritis. Involvement of the terminal interphalangeal joints of the fingers (Heberden's nodes) and of the first (thumb) carpometacarpal joint is characteristic of the familial type of osteoarthritis seen particularly in women.

side (referred via the obturator nerve). It can also be difficult to differentiate from lumbar spine problems. However, symptomatic osteoarthritis of the hip is unlikely without a reduction in the range of movement, particularly internal rotation (best tested with both hip and knee flexed to 90 degrees—Fig. 2.3) and some radiological changes. An occasional cause of confusion is trochanteric bursitis, in which there is localized tenderness just distal to the greater trochanter, and the pain is relieved by a local injection of lignocaine.

Symptomatic osteoarthritis of the hip joint is managed by regular analgesic/anti-inflammatory drugs, the application of local heat, and a spell of prone lying for ten to twenty minutes in bed each night (to prevent a flexion contracture). Once a significant limp develops, the patient should probably use a walking stick. The correct length is one which reaches to the top of the greater trochanter, or to the bend of the wrist when standing, and it should be held in the opposite hand. Many patients require instruction from a physiotherapist about how to walk with a stick, including negotiating stairs. It appears sensible—if feasible—to restrict activities which aggravate the pain, but the value of more

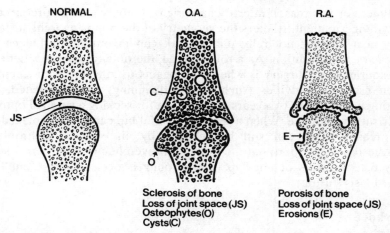

NORMAL   O.A.   R.A.

JS

C

O

E→

Sclerosis of bone
Loss of joint space (JS)
Osteophytes(O)
Cysts(C)

Porosis of bone
Loss of joint space (JS)
Erosions (E)

Fig. 2.2. Diagram illustrating the radiological changes in an osteoarthritic joint compared with those in a rheumatoid joint. Loss of joint space (actually loss of radiolucent articular cartilage) is a non-specific sign of joint damage. Osteophytes, cysts and periarticular osteosclerosis are the radiological signs of osteoarthritis. In the rheumatoid joint the characteristic changes are erosions and periarticular osteoporosis.

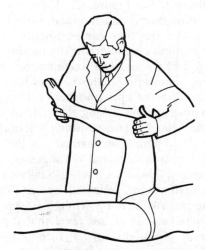

Fig. 2.3. Testing internal and external rotation of the hip joint.

complete rest is unproven. As exercise, cycling and swimming are usually better tolerated than weight-bearing activities.

Total prosthetic replacement has revolutionized the management of severe osteoarthritis of the hip. For the elderly it provides a complete answer to the problem. However, the younger the patient (below 60 years) the greater the chance that the replacement will fail within his lifetime. For this reason intertrochanteric osteotomy may be preferred in the younger patient. It alters the geometry of the opposing joint surfaces and, in a manner not fully understood, can favourably influence the course of the condition. As a rough guide, the time to refer a patient for consideration of surgery is when pain begins to interfere with sleep, or when essential activities (such as breadwinning) are threatened, but waiting lists of up to two years are a reason for seeking a surgical opinion early rather than late. When a severely painful hip cannot be replaced for any reason, pain can still be relieved by an excision arthroplasty (Girdlestone operation)—at the price of a severely unstable joint. Secondary osteoarthritis of one hip in the young is occasionally treated by arthrodesis (fusion).

The knee

Osteoarthritis of the knee is an extremely common cause of both troublesome minor symptoms and also serious disability. Lacking the deep ball-and-socket arrangement of the hip, it readily becomes unstable. Large effusions are usually obvious as horseshoe-shaped swellings above and down either side of the patella. Smaller effusions are detected by the three manoeuvres illustrated in Figure 2.4. There are two compartments to the knee: the patello-femoral and the main tibio-femoral articulation. Osteoarthritis may affect the two compartments to different degrees. Patello-femoral involvement characteristically produces pain on climbing stairs or rising from a chair and, on examination, rubbing the patella against the underlying femoral condyles is painful. A characteristic sign of this is elicited by holding the upper border of the patella firmly against the femur with one finger, then asking the patient to, 'press the knee down firmly onto the couch'. The resulting friction between the two surfaces produces a sharp pain. Osteoarthritis of the main compartment has to be differentiated from internal derangements such as meniscal lesions and loose bodies. These characteristically produce episodes of painful 'locking' or 'giving way', followed by an effusion which settles over a few days. The main knee compartment is opposite the mid-point of the patellar ligament, and is at this level that it may be possible to palpate the collateral ligaments or a torn meniscus. Knee joint examination should include an assessment of both lateral and antero-posterior stability (by the manoeuvres illustrated in Figure 2.5) and also

Fig. 2.4. Three manoeuvres for detecting fluid in the knee joint. (a) Eliciting cross-fluctuation between the upper and lower parts of the joint: a rapid method of detecting large effusions. (b) Patellar tap sign: suitable for detecting medium sized effusions. The examiner's left hand forces fluid from the large supra-patellar pouch into the main knee compartment, thus 'floating' the patella off the underlying femoral condyles. Pushing the patella posteriorly sharply using at least three

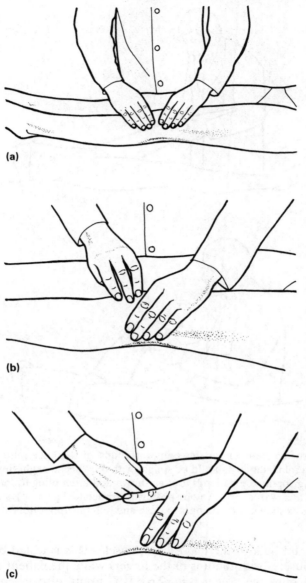

(a)

(b)

(c)

digits of the right hand then produces—if fluid is present—a characteristic tap as it strikes the condyles. (c) The bulge sign: suitable for detecting small effusions. The left hand again forces fluid out of the supra-patellar pouch, but here the index finger steadies the patella, while the fingers of the right hand stroke the groove between the patella and the femur—alternately on the medial and the lateral sides. Small effusions will be seen to bulge in this groove as the opposite side is stroked.

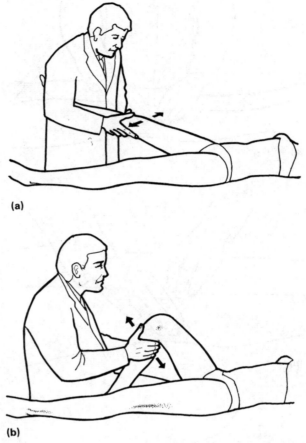

(a)

(b)

Fig. 2.5. Two manoeuvres for detecting instability of the knee joint. (a) Lateral stability. Lateral instability should be sought with the knee in slight flexion. This is achieved by gripping the patient's foot as shown and attempting to force the knee into valgus and varus. (b) Antero-posterior (cruciate ligament) stability. The examiner sits as shown and attempts to push and pull the upper tibia.

the power and bulk of the quadriceps muscle. This is tested by gripping the thigh muscles with the tips of the fingers while the patient presses his knee down onto the couch (Fig. 2.6). It is useful also to compare the circumference of the two thighs 20 cm above the upper border of the patella. The quadriceps muscles (the guardians of the knee joint) are the main stabilizers of the joint. Strengthening them by active exercises is an important aspect of physiotherapy.

The most common presentation of knee osteoarthritis in general practice is in an obese middle-aged patient. Examination is likely to

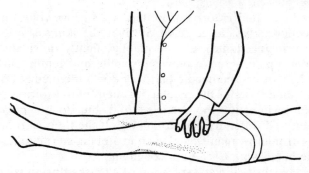

Fig. 2.6. Assessment of the quadriceps muscle. The examiner grips the quadriceps with the finger tips while the patient attempts to press the knee joint down onto the couch.

reveal a modest effusion, pain on extremes of movement and—most characteristic—crepitus. X-rays at this stage will probably show early osteophytes and perhaps some narrowing of one or other of the tibio-femoral compartments. The most important aspect of early management is indoctrination about the need for regular exercises to strengthen the quadriceps muscles. Advice alone (with or without a booklet) is not always enough. It requires sessions with a physiotherapist and follow-up to check that quadriceps power is being improved. Improving stability of the joint by exercise is often more effective than drug therapy at relieving pain. Nevertheless, most of these patients are prescribed a regular non-steroidal anti-inflammatory drug plus an analgesic to use as required. If pain is localized to one aspect of the knee, and a tender point can be identified, it may be worth infiltrating this area with 0.5 ml lignocaine (1 per cent) plus 0.5 ml of a corticosteroid preparation. Local heat from an infrared lamp, electric pad or hot water bottle can also provide useful pain relief.

More acute flares of arthritis (as shown by an effusion and warmth of the overlying skin) can be treated with an intra-articular injection of corticosteroid. The technique is relatively simple and can safely be done in the surgery provided that sterile disposable equipment and a careful 'no-touch' technique are employed.

Knee joint injection technique
With the patient lying on a couch and the leg in slight external rotation (and before washing the hands thoroughly) palpate the joint and plan the point of entry. Next 'scrub', then load a syringe with either hydrocortisone acetate 75 mg (3 ml) or triamcinolone hexacetonide 20 mg (1 ml). If inexperienced, or if any difficulty is anticipated, load another syringe with 2 ml lignocaine (1 per cent) (for a straightforward injection in experienced hands, local anaesthetic is best omitted). Use a 21 gauge

(green) needle if fluid is to be aspirated, a 23 gauge (blue) if a cortico-steroid injection only is to be given. Sterilize the skin (using a disposable sachet of sterilizing liquid), tip the patella slightly down on the lateral side (to open up the groove between patella and femur on the medial side—Fig. 2.7), insert the needle half way down the medial border of the patella, and slide it under the patella. It is helpful to aspirate any obvious effusion before injecting the corticosteroid, but do not persevere (and cause bleeding) if difficulty is encountered. If the fluid is to be examined for crystals or micro-organisms place it in a plain, sterile tube; if for cells, mix it immediately with EDTA anticoagulant.

In the osteoarthritic knee, aspiration of a tense effusion is always good practice. Injection of corticosteroid, however, should be regarded as a means of providing temporary relief (lasting days or weeks) when there is a troublesome flare. There is uncertainty about the effect of multiple corticosteroid injections on joint tissues. The authors would not exceed four such injections per year.

Instability of the osteoarthritic knee often leads to varus (bow leg) deformity. Owing to the altered line of weight transmission this is usually progressive and damaging. Management consists of restricting weight-bearing, the provision of a walking stick (or more supportive walking aid), quadriceps drill, anti-inflammatory/analgesic drugs and local warmth. Splinting is generally either ineffective or poorly tolerated. However, the Canadian (CARS-B) telescopic splint may occasionally be effective in counteracting a varus (or valgus) deformity while allowing knee flexion/extension. The detailed attention to fitting required for this is usually provided by Occupational Therapy Departments. For badly damaged knees in patients unsuitable for surgery, a hinged caliper and walking frame may allow movement about the house.

As at the hip, consideration of surgery may be indicated either because

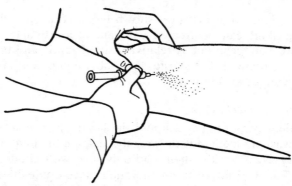

Fig. 2.7. Knee injection technique. The mid-point of the patella on the medial aspect is usually the easiest approach. A finger on the lateral border of the patella can tip it and thus open up the groove on the medial side.

of unacceptable pain (keeping the patient awake at night) or the threat of serious disability (such as loss of job or inability to do basic house work) or isolation. For those over 60 years of age total knee replacement is often the treatment of choice. With younger patients, especially if a varus or valgus deformity is associated with a good range of normal movement, some form of osteotomy (allowing correction of alignment) can be very useful. In a fit young patient with secondary osteoarthritis of one knee (and good hip and lumbar spine function) an arthrodesis (fusion) may be undertaken.

Heberden's nodes and osteoarthritis of the thumb carpometacarpal joint

Perhaps the most familiar image of osteoarthritis is the hand of the middle-aged or elderly woman affected by the primary osteoarthritis which runs in families (Fig. 2.8). This hand involvement may or may not be associated with osteoarthritis elsewhere.

Although the split-pea-sized, bony-hard Heberden's nodes at the base of the terminal phalanx are highly characteristic, they nevertheless have to be differentiated from gouty tophi and psoriatic arthritis. They often occur independently of thumb carpometacarpal joint involvement, and vice versa. Usually Heberden's nodes are no more than unsightly, and the doctor's responsibility is to reassure the patient that she does not have rheumatoid arthritis. Rarely, cystic degeneration of the cartilage cap of a

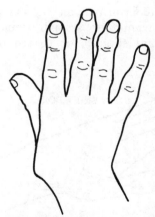

Fig. 2.8. The familial pattern of osteoarthritis in the hand. This pattern of joint involvement is more common in women. The osteophytes at the base of the terminal phalanges are Heberden's nodes. Involvement of the first carpometacarpal joint of the thumb gives the hand a square outline due to (a) bony swelling of the joint, (b) adduction deformity of the metacarpal, and (c) wasting of the nearby small muscles.

node may produce acute local inflammation. Aspiration and injection of a small quantity of corticosteroid can produce considerable relief.

Osteoarthritis of the thumb carpometacarpal joint produces a characteristic 'square hand' appearance (Fig. 2.8), due to a combination of bony swelling, local muscle wasting, plus an adduction deformity of the metacarpal. This lesion can be both painful and disabling, and is often wrongly diagnosed as rheumatoid arthritis. Fortunately, an intra-articular injection of corticosteroid can produce dramatic relief of pain, and this may last for weeks or even months. An alternative method of treatment is to use a working splint which leaves the interphalangeal joint of the thumb free to move.

Technique for injecting the thumb carpometacarpal joint

The joint forms the distal border of the anatomical snuff box (Fig. 2.9). Place a palpating finger over the base of the metacarpal while, with the other hand, apply intermittent traction to the thumb. The palpating finger should be able to feel the joint opening and closing. Palpate also the radial artery as it crosses the joint. Once the anatomy is identified, 'scrub', sterilize the skin, then—while exerting traction on the thumb—'feel' the tip of a 23 gauge needle into the joint (avoiding the radial artery) and inject about 0.2 ml of a corticosteroid suspension.

GENERAL PRINCIPLES OF MANAGEMENT IN OSTEOARTHRITIS

Most patients with osteoarthritis can be managed satisfactorily by the primary health care team. Only a small proportion will have disease severe enough to warrant surgery, or to require the resources of a specialist department.

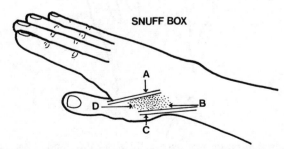

Fig. 2.9. The anatomical snuff box. The proximal border of this rectangular area consists of the styloid process of the radius (B), the distal border is the first carpometacarpal joint (D), the palmar border is the tendon of abductor pollicis longus (C), the dorsal border is the tendon of extensor pollicis longus (A), while the floor (shaded) is the scaphoid bone.

Explanation

Time needs to be spent with the patient to explain the nature of the condition. Patients need to understand that there are irreversible changes in the joints, but that painful episodes tend to be temporary, and the condition may progress only very gradually. The limitations of drug therapy and the role of surgery need to be clarified at this stage so that unrealistic expectations are not fostered. The doctor needs to understand the patient's fears about the condition ('Will I end up in a wheel chair?' 'Arthritis means I am getting old.') and patient and doctor together need to plan some realistic objectives for management.

Pain relief

This is considered in detail in Chapter 17. Patients often have over-optimistic expectations of what drug therapy can achieve. The most that can be expected is a modest background of pain relief with regular non-steroidal anti-inflammatory therapy and additional analgesics to cope with episodic bad patches. It is worth experimenting with one or two anti-inflammatories because individual metabolism of these drugs varies widely. However, it is important to avoid bolstering unrealistic expectations by trying preparation after preparation and giving the patient the impression that the 'perfect drug' will eventually be found. Pain can often be eased by the use of simple home remedies such as hot baths or the application of local heat by a hot water bottle, electric pad or sunlamp. Rubifacients and massage can also be comforting and provide temporary analgesia on a counter-irritation principle, although it should be clearly explained that these measures do not influence the course of the condition.

Pain relief may also be achieved by looking at wider aspects of the patient's lifestyle and environment. Losing weight and attention to care of the feet may allow an osteoarthritic patient to get out of the house again. The physiotherapist has an important role to play, both in pain relief and in bringing about change in the patient's way of life. She may be asked to plan a specific programme of active, resisted exercises to strengthen muscles acting across a diseased joint. This in itself may produce pain relief. In addition, the community physiotherapist, seeing the patients in their own homes, is in the best position to advise on appropriate walking aids and train patients in their use. While in the home they may also be able to advise on small changes in the patient's environment which will improve functional ability. For example, shifting the furniture around, advising on the position of rails, and supervising practice in negotiating stairs, may give an elderly patient the confidence to remain at home with less fear of falling. However, physiotherapy is a scarce resource, and it is important to keep in mind the therapeutic objective of each referral. It is also important that doctors and patients bear in mind that the specific techniques of physiotherapists such as ultrasound or heat give only short-term pain relief, while their educational function may enable the patients to carry on with exercises and activities at home with lasting benefit. Combining all these aspects of pain control makes the patient feel that appropriate attention is being directed towards his condition, and an increased sense of well-being may contribute to improved pain relief.

Self-help groups

Patients should be encouraged to join self-help groups. These provide education about the condition, ideas for solving practical problems, and a club for social events. The Arthritis and Rheumatism Council produces useful educational literature for patients. A list of available topics is to be found in Appendix 3.

Aids and appliances

More severely disabled patients may require the occupational therapist to visit them at home to assess whether any aids, appliances or home adaptions may be necessary. A social worker may be of value to help patients sort out which allowances they may be eligible for.

SPONDYLOSIS

Degenerative joint disease of the spine affects both the main (anterior) intervertebral joints and also the facetal (posterior, apophyseal) articulations. The facetal joint changes are exactly comparable to osteoarthritis in other joints. In the anterior joints the intervertebral discs play an important role in determining the pattern of spondylosis.

The anatomical relationships of the discs and the vertebrae are shown diagrammatically in Figure 2.10. Proteoglycans in the semi-liquid nucleus pulposus attract water, causing the nucleus to swell and create tension within the confines of the limiting annulus fibrosus. This 'spring-loaded cushion' acts as an effective shock absorber while allowing some spinal movement.

The intervertebral disc is susceptible to two common forms of pathological change. The first is herniation (prolapse, protrusion), in which mechanical stress produces either a rupture of the annulus, allowing outward (horizontal) herniation of the nucleus, or vertical herniation of the nucleus through the cartilagenous endplate into the body of the vertebra, to give the familiar appearance of a Schmorl's node on X-ray (Fig. 2.11). The second change is shrinkage of the discs with ageing, due

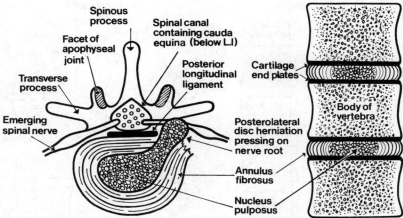

Fig. 2.10. Vertical and lateral diagrams of a lumbar vertebra. On the left is indicated the route taken by a postero-lateral disc herniation. Note how the emerging spinal nerve roots lie between the discs anteriorly and the facetal (apophyseal) joints posteriorly. They are thus liable to compression by both disc protrusions and bony osteophytes.

to loss of proteoglycan from the nucleus. This is reflected in disc space narrowing on X-ray, and is a cause of loss of body height in the elderly.

Mechanical factors tend to direct horizontal disc protrusions posteriorly. However, the strong posterior longitudinal ligament deflects them postero-laterally. The implications of this will be clear from consideration of Figure 2.10. Each spinal nerve root, as it emerges, lies in the pathway both of a postero-lateral disc protrusion and of osteophytes from the facetal joint. Hence it is that—both in the cervical and the lumbar regions—disc lesions and spondylosis tend to produce pain both locally and down the related limb (brachial neuralgia and sciatica).

Degenerative changes in the vertebral bodies are reflected in the formation of osteophytes. These develop at the vertebral rim and grow outwards, often in a beaked shape ('parrot-beak' osteophytes—Fig. 2.11). This pattern suggests that the stimulus to their formation may be a disc protrusion which, by elevating the periosteum from the vertebral body, causes new bone to be laid down round the protrusion. These various bone changes produce a highly characteristic appearance on X-ray. They are illustrated diagrammatically in Figure 2.11. Occasionally, inwardly directed bony overgrowth may combine with disc protrusions to produce *spinal canal stenosis*.

The discussion of spondylosis and disc lesions applies equally to the cervical and the lumbar regions of the spine (thoracic lesions are relatively rare). However, there are two obvious and important differences. At the cervical level any protrusion into the spinal canal will lead

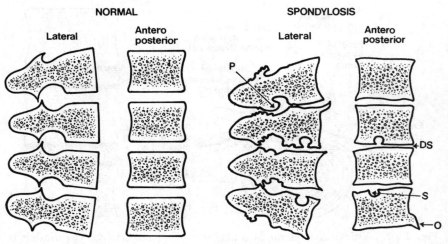

Fig. 2.11. Diagrams of lateral and antero-posterior X-rays of lumbar vertebrae to contrast the appearances of normal and spondylotic spines. The characteristic changes include loss of height of disc spaces (DS), osteophytes (O) arising from the edges of the vertebrae (the upper border of the second vertebra down in the lateral view illustrates a typical 'parrot-beak' osteophyte), and Schmorl's nodes (S) indicating the site of vertical herniations into the bodies of the vertebrae. In addition, outgrowths of osteophytes (P) from the facetal (apophyseal) joints may protrude into the intervertebral notch and there press on the emerging nerve roots.

to a myelopathy (with long tract signs and extensor plantar responses); but, because the spinal cord ends at the level of L_1, lumbar lesions which extend into the canal will press on the *cauda equina* to produce lower motor neurone signs. The other difference is that the vertebral artery travels up through foramina in the cervical vertebrae. Cervical spondylosis can thus cause vertebro-basilar insufficiency (with vertigo on looking upwards).

From the above description it will be clear that vertebral and disc lesions are closely linked, and that disc lesion may range from acute mechanical derangements to chronic degenerative changes. The bony lesions are dramatically obvious on X-ray (Fig. 2.11), but disc protrusions require special imaging techniques (radiculography or CT scanning) to identify them.

The clinical manifestations of degenerative joint disease affecting the cervical and lumbar spines are discussed in Chapters 10 and 11.

REFERENCES

Buchanan, W. W. and Dick, W. C. (1983). Osteoarthrosis. In *Rheumatic Diseases:*

Collected Reports 1959–1983. (ed. C. F. Hawkins and H. L. F. Currey). The Arthritis and Rheumatism Council, London.

Gardner, D. L. (1983). The nature and causes of osteoarthrosis. *Br. med. J.* **286**, 418–24.

Nuki, G. (ed) (1980). *The aetiopathogenesis of osteoarthrosis.* Pitman Medical, London.

Office of Population Censuses and Surveys (1979). *Morbidity statistics from general practice: Second national study 1971–1972.* HMSO, London.

Sokoloff, L. (ed) (1985). Osteoarthritis. *Clinics in Rheumatic Diseases* **11**, (2). W. B. Saunders, London.

3 Inflammatory joint disease I:

Rheumatoid arthritis

Rheumatoid arthritis is the most common cause of inflammatory joint disease. Although it usually presents with arthritis, it is a systemic disease with a wide variety of extra-articular manifestations. For this reason rheumatoid is included amongst the systemic connective tissue disorders.

Epidemiology

Population surveys in several countries show a prevalence rate of between 1 per cent and 2 per cent, with the peak age of onset in the fifth decade of life (Fig. 3.1). This is probably an underestimate, and there is some evidence from X-ray surveys that a number of people have asymptomatic rheumatoid changes in their joints. Rheumatoid factor occurs in about 5 per cent of the population, a prevalence much higher than that of rheumatoid disease (2 per cent). It is also present in a number of other conditions, and in a small proportion of the normal population. (See Appendix 1 for details of tests and their interpretation.)

The spectrum of the disease is very wide and, contrary to its popular image, only a third of patients progress to persistent disabling disease.

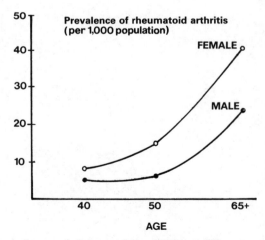

Fig. 3.1. The prevalance of rheumatoid arthritis at different ages. This demonstrates that women are affected three times as often as men, and that amongst the elderly rheumatoid is a common condition.

28

Furthermore, only about 10 per cent become so disabled that they require a wheelchair. It is impossible to make an accurate prediction about the course of the disease in an individual with rheumatoid arthritis. In general, women tend to have more severe disease than men. However, the uncommon but severe extra-articular features occur mainly amongst men. Pointers to a less favourable prognosis include:

Insidious onset of the disease.
Persistent activity without remission beyond a year.
Extra-articular manifestations, particularly vasculitis.
Strongly positive tests for rheumatoid factor.

The disease process

The cause of rheumatoid arthritis is still unknown, but the pathological processes which lead to inflammation and joint destruction are becoming clearer. The central event within the joint cavity is the combination of antibodies and antigens to produce immune complexes. These trigger the cascade of enzymes in the complement pathway and attract poly-morphonuclear leucocytes. These phagocytose the immune complexes and, in so doing, release lysosomal enzymes and other mediators of inflammation. Continued stimulation of the synovial lining by these chemical mediators of inflammation eventually leads to an outgrowth of granulation tissue (pannus). Cells within the pannus release enzymes which are able to digest both cartilage and bone. This enables the pannus to invade the joint cartilage and penetrate into the underlying bone producing the erosions characteristic of rheumatoid arthritis. These changes can be seen on X-rays as loss of joint space (loss of cartilage) and bone erosions, which may eventually destroy the bone ends. Similar pathological changes occur in any of the inflammatory arthritides, and a synovial biopsy will not show changes specific to rheumatoid arthritis.

What initiates and maintains this process is unknown, nor is the role of the autoantibody rheumatoid factor understood. Rheumatoid arthritis is classed as an autoimmune disorder, and—as in other such conditions—there is evidence of an immunological aberration in which the control, by T-cells, of immunological responsiveness is defective, allowing the expression of inappropriate immune reactivity, including reactivity against 'self' antigens. A chronic virus infection of T-cells is one possible explanatory hypothesis for this phenomenon. Patients with rheumatoid arthritis have an excess of the tissue antigen HLA-DR4, which suggests that genetic factors play some part. Opinions differ about the role of rheumatoid factors. These are antibodies directed against immuno-globulin G (IgG), in other words, 'anti-antibodies' (see Appendix 1). Some regard IgG itself as the central antigen involved, others consider the presence of rheumatoid factor as an epiphenomenon in the rheumatoid process, or at most as playing a contributory role in the formation of immune complexes. (Whatever its pathological role, its diagnostic value is great.) For a full discussion of the immunological aspects of rheumatoid arthritis see *Clinics in Rheumatic Disease* (1986).

Initial clinical presentation

GPs often see patients at a very early stage in an illness, when a number of symptoms may not yet fit any recognized diagnostic category. For example, it is a common experience that only in retrospect can one fit a frozen shoulder or a painful foot into the emerging picture of rheumatoid disease. The difficulty for the doctor is in deciding who to investigate, and when to start the process. The most useful clinical pointers to rheumatoid arthritis are a history of early morning stiffness and the presence of joint swelling and tenderness. The appropriate screening tests in these circumstances are the ESR and latex test. The use of time as a diagnostic tool, in combination with regular clinical review, is particularly useful.

It is a mistake to do extensive laboratory investigations too early: they are commonly un-informative, only supporting the clinical diagnosis of an early polyarthritis. In particular, early X-rays are of little diagnostic value, although they may form a valuable baseline from which to assess later changes. They may also be reassuring to the patient. Symptomatic relief with analgesics or non-steroidal anti-inflammatory drugs will be the most appropriate treatment until the diagnosis is clear.

Usually rheumatoid arthritis presents in one of the four ways listed below. Rarely it presents with extra-articular manifestations such as Sjøgren's syndrome, or lung nodules found on a routine chest X-ray which mimic secondaries. (See Table 3.1 for a list of extra-articular features).

1. Symmetrical polyarthritis

Susan, 28, complained of increasing joint pain over the past six weeks with stiffness in the hands, feet and shoulders. She needed a hot bath every morning to loosen up, and ached after sitting still. Examination showed spindling of the fingers, a 'boggy' swelling in the metacarpophalangeal joints, and pain on squeezing the metatarsophalangeal joints. There was slight tenderness in the left knee, but no effusion. Investigations revealed: ESR 50 mm/hour, Hb 12.2 g/dl, latex test negative, anti-nuclear antibody (ANA) negative. X-rays of the hands showed slight local osteoporosis only.

At this stage there is quite a wide differential to consider. Although the clinical picture suggests rheumatoid arthritis other possibilities could be: seronegative rheumatoid arthritis; virus infections (e.g. rubella, mumps, hepatitis, glandular fever); systemic lupus erythematosis (SLE); sero-negative spondarthritidies; rheumatic fever; reactive arthritis.

Susan was treated with non-steroidal anti-inflammatory drugs and her joint symptoms settled over two months. A year later they recurred; her latex test was now positive. She remained well controlled on non-steroidal anti-inflammatory drugs.

2. Monoarthritis

Lilly, 78, had had 'rheumatism' in her left elbow for years, for which she had used paracetamol and never bothered her GP. She came to show him a lump which had recently developed. This was a classical rheumatoid nodule. X-rays showed severe erosive changes at the elbow, but nowhere else. She remained on paracetamol, which suited her best.

3. Systemic upset with widespread stiffness

Mrs White, 68, requested a visit. She had been in bed for three days aching all over. She had a cold. Her GP thought she had the 'flu' and suggested paracetamol and bed rest. Another visit a week later, when she was still confined to bed stiff and aching, revealed a swollen knee and tenderness of the wrists and hands. ESR 55 mm/hour, latex 1 in 80. She did not respond well to indomethacin and later required D-penicillamine.

4. Palindromic rheumatism

John, a 52-year-old messenger, attended the doctor's surgery to report an episode of severe pain in the left shoulder. It had lasted about twelve hours, but had now settled. Examination was normal. A month later he required a visit for a painful knee. He said it was red and swollen, but it had settled before the doctor arrived. Over the next six months he had three further episodes of pain lasting six to eight hours, which were helped a little by naproxen. X-rays and blood tests showed no abnormality. His GP began to wonder whether his symptoms were due to anxiety, but some months later he was admitted to hospital following the rupture of a Baker's cyst behind his right knee. The latex test was positive and he had early erosions on hand and foot X-rays.

Palindromic rheumatism (severe, episodic joint pains, lasting a few hours or days) is not common. Fifty per cent of patients will continue to have episodic attacks, about 35 per cent will develop rheumatoid arthritis and the remaining 15 per cent may remit. A few will develop SLE.

CLINICAL FEATURES OF JOINT DISEASE

Rheumatoid arthritis typically presents as a symmetrical polyarthritis affecting the small and medium-sized joints (Fig. 3.2). Apart from the cervical spine, the back is rarely affected, and patients with back pain should be suspected of having one of the spondarthritides (see Chapter

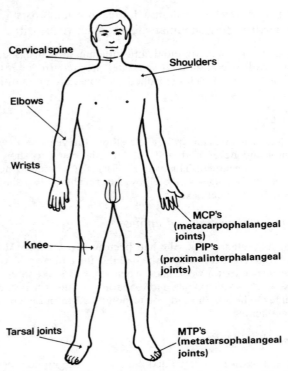

Cervical spine

Shoulders

Elbows

Wrists

MCP's (metacarpophalangeal joints)

Knee

PIP's (proximalinterphalangeal joints)

Tarsal joints

MTP's (metatarsophalangeal joints)

Fig. 3.2. The distribution of affected joints in rheumatoid arthritis.

4). The terminal interphalangeal joints are also spared; involvement of these would suggest osteoarthritis or psoriatic arthritis.

Symptoms and signs

The most common presenting complaints are those of joint pain, prolonged early morning stiffness, and loss of function. The joint pain is experienced as a constant ache, made worse by putting pressure on the joint. Inflamed hands may present as feeling swollen, or weak, or as the loss of ability to do accustomed tasks such as knitting or unscrewing jars. Patients with irritable metatarsophalangeal joints often feel as though they are walking on small pebbles or broken glass. Early signs may include an inability to make a full fist, or loss of full elevation at the shoulders. Joint tenderness is best assessed by gently squeezing across the joint while passively moving it (Fig. 3.3(a)), and by noting tenderness at the extremes of range.

Morning stiffness is highly characteristic of all inflammatory arthropathies. It can often last several hours and be very disabling. It may be

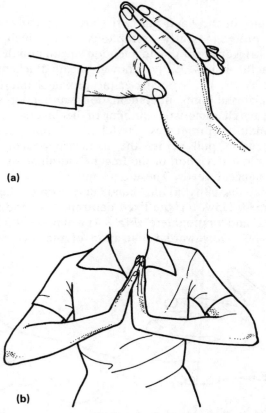

Fig. 3.3. (a) Assessing joint tenderness by gentle squeezing across the metacarpo-phalangeal joints. (b) Demonstrating loss of dorsiflexion in the right wrist.

difficult to describe. Instead one may get reports of the patient's response to it: 'I have to get up two hours earlier to get going', 'It takes me an hour to get dressed. My husband has to get the kids up.' Some are helped by a hot bath or by running their hands under hot or cold water. The stiffness will recur in the day if the joints are not kept moving.

As the arthritis progresses, irreversible damage to the joints occurs. Effusions and synovial hypertrophy stretch the joint capsule which may lead to subluxation and instability. Weakness of the surrounding muscles due to pain, disuse or neuropathy adds to the problem. As the cartilage and bone are destroyed the joints may develop fixed deformities. A patient who is no longer showing evidence of active inflammation may still have considerable joint pain and loss of function due to the mechanical disruption of joints.

The hand

The small joints in the hand and wrist are frequently affected by the rheumatoid process. Early symptoms may include Raynaud's phenomenon, trigger finger due to a tendon sheath nodule, or a sensation of fullness in the hands. Early synovial sheath thickening may cause carpel tunnel syndrome. Synovitis at the proximal interphalangeal and metacarpophalangeal joints, in combination with tendon sheath involvement, will cause a characteristic spindling of the fingers.

As the condition progresses, stretching of the joint capsule and unbalanced tendon pull across the metacarpophalangeal joints will contribute to ulnar deviation of the fingers and ulnar subluxation of the metacarpophalangeal heads. These deformities often cause surprisingly little functional disability to the hand, and correct themselves as an object is grasped. However, the fixed deformities of the fingers such as the 'swan-neck' and 'boutonniere' (Fig. 3.4) will prevent fist formation—a serious disability. Downward subluxation of the metacarpophalangeal

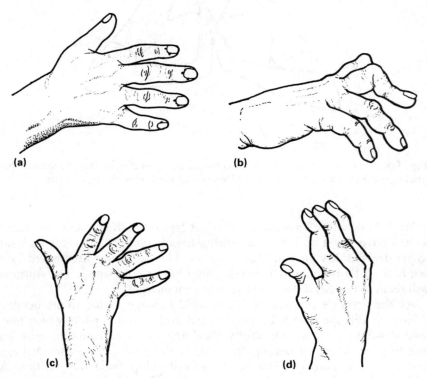

(a)

(b)

(c)

(d)

Fig. 3.4. Hand deformities in rheumatoid arthritis. (a) Spindling of the fingers and nail-fold vasculitis. (b) Boutonniere finger deformity. (c) Ulnar deviation with metacarpophalangeal joint subluxation. (d) Swan-neck finger deformity.

joints and tendon rupture, causing finger drop, also pose a serious threat to useful hand function.

The knee

Involvement of the knee joint is common. Serious damage at this joint is the most significant factor in confining rheumatoid patients to a wheel-chair, so early management is important. Joint tenderness and effusion are common early signs, and draining the fluid may give dramatic relief of pain. Steroid can be injected locally three of four times in a year. This usually gives only transient relief, but may tide the patient through a crisis. As the capsule is stretched, a Baker's cyst may form behind the knee. Occasionally the synovial membrane ruptures and the fluid tracks down the calf, causing an inflamed swollen leg which is difficult to distinguish from a deep vein thrombosis. Synovitis of the knee is painful, and patients frequently rest with a pillow under the knee. This position encourages flexion contractures which must be avoided if the patient is to remain mobile. As the joint surface is damaged a valgus (or less commonly a varus) deformity may develop, and in time this may become unstable. Continued weight-bearing on an unbalanced joint will tend to increase the deformity (Fig. 3.5). This can be helped by splinting or by surgery.

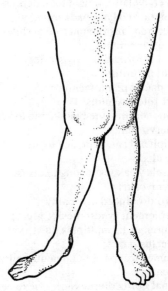

Fig. 3.5. Valgus deformity of the knee.

Extra-articular features of rheumatoid arthritis

As rheumatoid arthritis is a generalized systemic disease it is not unusual to find manifestations outside the joints. Some of these extra-articular features are listed in Table 3.1. When the disease is in an active phase it is often accompanied by a low-grade fever, a general feeling of illness, lethargy and weakness, and a widespread lymphadenopathy. It is hardly surprising that depression is frequently encountered in the face of chronic pain, loss of the ability to do normal activities, and an uncertain future. Of the commoner extra-articular manifestations carpal tunnel syndrome needs special mention. It is frequently found in association with rheumatoid and the combination of articular and neurological deficit can prove disastrous for hand function. The diagnosis is frequently missed. Patients should be routinely asked about numbness and tingling in the fingers and electrical conduction studies should be obtained if doubt remains about the diagnosis. Treatment is straightforward, (splinting, local steroid injection or surgery), and can greatly improve hand function for a patient. (See Chapter 13 for further details.)

Table 3.1. *Extra-articular features of rheumatoid arthritis (including some effects of drug treatment)*

General:	Fever, malaise, weight loss, depression
	Generalized lymphadenopathy
	Subcutaneous rheumatoid nodules
Tendons and bursae:	Tenosynovitis
	Nodule formation 'trigger finger'
	Tendon rupture
Vasculitis:	Raynaud's phenomenon
	Nail-fold vasculitis
	Mononeuritis (see below) due to vasculitis in the vasa nervorum
	Peripheral gangrene due to arterial occlusion
	Leg ulcers
Muscle:	Muscle weakness owing to disuse
	Polymyositis
	Steroid-induced myopathy
Nervous system:	Entrapment syndromes, (e.g. carpal tunnel, ulnar neuritis)
	Mononeuritis multiplex due to vasa nervorum occlusion
	Symmetrical peripheral neuropathy, either motor or sensory
	Spinal-cord compression, due to cervical spine involvement

Table 3.1. *Continued*

Eyes:	Keratoconjunctivitis sicca, as part of Sjøgren's syndrome
	Scleritis, occasionally proceeding to scleromalacia perforans
The heart:	Pericarditis
	Endocarditis
	Post-mortem finding of nodules in the heart or pericardium
The lungs:	Pleural effusion
	Fibrosing alveolitis
	Lung nodules
	Caplan's syndrome (pneumoconiosis, rheumatoid arthritis, and large pulmonary nodules)
	Bronchiolitis
Renal:	Amyloid disease
	Immune-complex nephrosis secondary to gold/penicillamine therapy
	Interstitial nephritis owing to non-steroidal anti-inflammatory drugs
Haematological:	Iron-deficiency anaemia
	Anaemia of chronic disease
	Hypersplenism as part of Felty's syndrome
	Marrow suppression following treatment with gold or penicillamine
	Macrocytic anaemia, possibly due to folate deficiency
	Haemolytic anaemia

Diagnosis and investigation

Diagnostic criteria

In 1959 the American Rheumatism Association drew up a method for the diagnosis of rheumatoid arthritis by which eight clinical and pathological criteria were used to divide cases into 'classical', 'definite' or 'probable'. Although internationally recognized, these criteria have become less used, especially with recent advances in the understanding of the seronegative arthropathies. In practice a diagnosis of rheumatoid arthritis is made by grouping together clinical and laboratory findings. These consist of: symmetrical inflammatory polyarthritis with a typical pattern of joint involvement; subcutaneous nodules (only found in 25 per cent of cases); positive rheumatoid factor tests; erosive changes on X-rays.

About 15 per cent of patients with otherwise typical rheumatoid disease remain seronegative. It is important to exclude other causes of polyarthritis in this group, but once this is done management is the same as for those with seropositive rheumatoid arthritis.

Haematology

The ESR is usually raised. It reflects inflammatory activity, and is usually a good marker of disease activity. Anaemia is generally present (see below) and there is often an increased white cell count and thrombocythaemia. This reflects marrow hyperactivity.

Immunological tests

IgM rheumatoid factors are not a specific test for rheumatoid arthritis. They are found in about 85 per cent of patients with the condition, but they are also associated with a number of other chronic diseases and are found in about 5 per cent of the normal population (see Appendix 1). In spite of these caveats, finding a positive rheumatoid factor is the most useful diagnostic test available and the early appearance of a high titre of rheumatoid factor correlates positively with a severe form of the arthritis. Positive tests for anti-nuclear antibody and lupus erythematosus cells occur in about 20 per cent of patients with rheumatoid arthritis, but only in those with rheumatoid factor.

Radiology

Early films may show non-specific changes of an inflammatory arthropathy. These include soft tissue shadows and peri-articular osteoporosis. Later changes reflect the destruction of articular cartilage and bone. There will be narrowing of the joint space and erosive changes (see Fig. 2.2 p. 15). These are 'bites' out of the surface of the bone, which always communicate with the joint cavity. Erosions are most commonly seen in films of the hands and feet. These are the best films with which to monitor the disease process.

TREATMENT OF RHEUMATOID ARTHRITIS

Since the cause of rheumatoid arthritis remains unknown and prevention is not yet possible, treatment of the symptoms of the disease remains an empirical process, and predicting the response to treatment for any individual is a hazardous business. Untreated, the disease runs a fluctuating course with relapses and remissions. Owing to this it is easy to make claims for treatments which are in fact no better than placebo. Many of the established treatment regimens for rheumatoid arthritis carry considerable hazard to the patient and require them to have regular blood and urine checks.

Place of treatment

Advice on where the patient is best managed cannot be straightforward. It will vary according to the severity of the patient's illness, the interest and expertise of the GP, and the local rheumatological facilities. It is difficult for the GP to manage a case effectively if there is no open access to physiotherapy or occupational therapy, and no regular liaison with a rheumatology department; on the other hand some patients get frustrated attending a clinic which is difficult to reach, or in which they rarely see the same doctor.

In a chronic disease such as rheumatoid arthritis, probably the best solution is for the initial management and regular follow-up to be managed by the GP, with consultant opinions at particular key points in the decision-making process. This might involve using a 'shared-care' booklet for ease of communication, or the consultant making occasional visits to local practices. Regular review by a consultant could be confined to those patients with unusual problems. The scheme below outlines a 'stepped' approach to the management of rheumatoid arthritis.

Treatment of the disease	Treatment of the patient and modification of the environment
STAGE 1	
Non-steroidal anti-inflammatory drug treatment (other analgesia when required)	Explanation of the disease Counselling the patient and her family
Local steroid injections	Physiotherapy and advice on regular exercises
Monitoring the disease process	Occupational therapy advice on home aids Introduction to self-help groups
STAGE 2	
Introduction of a long-acting drug, e.g. gold or D- penicillamine	Physiotherapy for splints and exercises
Monitoring the disease process, and drug effects	Occupational therapy, advice on home adaptations
Treating other disease manifestations, e.g. anaemia, carpal tunnel syndrome, Sjøgren's	Chiropody Disabled car sticker

Treatment of the disease	Treatment of the patient and modification of the environment
STAGE 3	
Surgery to joints	Introduction of a wheelchair
Neurological complications	Involve social services for advice on:
Introduction of systemic steroids	Attendance allowance
	Mobility allowance
	Home help
Severe systemic disease	Meals-on-wheels
with vasculitis or other	Bath attendant
extra-articular manifestations	Holidays for the disabled

In practice many GPs are prepared to manage the disease at stage 1, some GPs will continue to supervise at stage 2, and all GPs need specialist advice at stage 3.

Many GPs will be uncertain how long to continue management at stage 1 because they are not sure about the criteria for shifting to a stage 2 approach. To make a sensible decision about this, a straightforward method of assessing the progress of the disease is needed as well as criteria for introducing the next stage of management. Clinicians vary considerably in the way they assess a patient, and the weight they put on laboratory or clinical findings. In practice it will be an amalgam of the following data:

The patient's report on how she feels.
A measure of the functional ability of the patient.
The extent of early morning stiffness.
An assessment of the number of joints actively inflamed.
Radiological evidence of the progression of erosive changes.
Laboratory indices, ESR, haemoglobin, rheumatoid factor.

Using some or all of these criteria it is possible to decide with the patient at each visit whether her condition is better, worse or the same. This process is greatly aided by seeing a regular doctor, and structuring the notes in some way (see Chapter 1). Further details of ways of assessing the amount of disability, and the extent of joint involvement can be found in Appendix 2.

Different clinicians vary in their timing of a decision to start someone on 'slow-acting' drugs (gold, penicillamine, azathioprine). The following are general guidelines.

1. Failure of non-steroidal anti-inflammatory drugs to give adequate symptomatic relief.
2. Persistent swollen joints with active synovitis over several months.
3. Progressive erosive changes over six months or so. (Hence the importance of hand and foot X-rays early on, to form a baseline for later comparison.)

In general, slow-acting drugs should be considered for anyone with definite rheumatoid disease which is erosive and progressive.

Drug treatment will be covered in detail in Chapter 16. Some of these decision points, and details of management, can best be illustrated by a case history.

Miss Dent, 55, takes thyroxine replacement for primary myxoedema. In 1979 she developed a frozen shoulder which lasted four months, and was treated with physiotherapy and two intra-articular steroid injections. In 1981 she came with two weeks pain in the right forefoot; the metatarsophalangeal joints were warm and tender to pressure.

The following differential was considered: gout; trauma, or a March fracture; inflammatory arthritis.

She was given indomethacin 50 mg b.d. while an X-ray, urate, ESR, and latex test were obtained. Apart from an ESR of 35 mm/hour all tests were normal, her painful foot eased on the tablets, but never really settled.

Three months later she attended with pain in the hands and early morning stiffness. Examination showed tenderness at the wrists, metacarpophalangeal and proximal interphalangeal joints, and some restriction of range of both shoulders. Her symptoms had spread to become a generalized inflammatory arthropathy.

The following diagnoses were considered: rheumatoid arthritis; SLE; psoriatic arthritis; reactive arthritis.

X-rays of her hands and feet showed no erosions; the ANA was negative; ESR 65 mm/hour, Hb 10.6 g/dl with a normochromic picture; the latex test was now positive at a titre of 1:80. She started indomethacin again, was seen by the physiotherapist to learn 'joint preservation exercises' and joined the British Rheumatism and Arthritis Association to find out about her condition. She said she had a brother with rheumatoid arthritis whose disease had gone into remission after a year.

Over a period of six months she developed ulnar deviation of the fingers and could no longer make a fist. She regularly had three hours morning stiffness, her feet were painful, and a nodule developed on her elbow. Referral to the community occupational therapist produced some useful kitchen aids for turning taps and opening jars. By this time she had reached the point where the introduction of a slow-acting drug should be considered, but she did not want to start any 'stronger medication', feeling that she could get on top of the condition herself.

At this stage in the illness, when a major treatment change is contemplated, it is important to review an objective record of the disease process with the patient. An assessment of the extent of the functional disability should be made, and the advantages and risks of more intensive treatment discussed. Many GPs will involve a consultant rheumatologist at this stage; those GPs with a special interest will institute 'phase 2' treatment with a slow-acting drug, with all the necessary blood and urine tests.

Repeat X-rays of Miss Dent's hands and feet now showed erosive changes; ESR 95 mm/hour, Hb 9.5 gm/dl. She eventually agreed to a trial of D-penicillamine, having first been warned that it could take up to three months to show an effect. It was started at a dose of 125 mg o.d., with fortnightly blood counts. She was prescribed Albustix and checked her own urine for protein. Over a period of two months the dose was increased to 500 mg a day, she lost her sense of taste and felt little better on the drug. Her anaemia was investigated, and showed a mixed microcytic and normocytic picture, with a low serum iron and total iron-binding capacity. Iron was prescribed but her haemoglobin did not rise above 10 g/dl. She became miserable and began to give up hope, even failing to attend physiotherapy. She took extra indomethacin to help the stiffness and developed dizziness until this was stopped.

At this point a specialist rheumatological opinion was requested. A domiciliary visit was arranged, in particular to consider a change of slow-acting drug. Both patient and GP gained useful support and advice from the consultation.

It was agreed that she should change to gold. This was introduced with weekly test doses of 10 mg and 20 mg followed by regular weekly injections of 50 mg. After about six weeks she began to improve. There was less morning stiffness, she could walk better and do more about the house. Her haemoglobin rose and her ESR fell to 35 mm/hour.

She became established on regular monthly gold injections (50 mg intramuscularly), but then developed a skin rash. This was a scaly eczematous reaction on her fingertips, arms, buttocks and chest. The gold injections were stopped, and she was referred to the skin department for advice on whether this was a gold reaction. Unfortunately she had a long wait, the eruption almost settled, and the dermatologist was uncertain but advised gradual re-introduction of the gold. During the wait her symptoms had returned, but settled again when the gold was restarted. These injections will be continued monthly as long as they benefit her.

Over the two years of disease activity her feet had been severely affected (Fig. 3.6). There was disruption of the subtalar joints with a valgus deformity; synovitis at the metatarsophalangeal joints had caused spreading of the forefoot and flattening of the longitudinal arch.

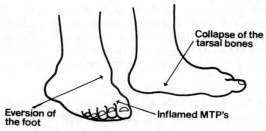

Fig. 3.6. Foot deformity in rheumatoid arthritis. Collapse of the tarsus with eversion of the foot, and 'dropping' of the metatarsophalangeal joints such that they take excessive weight.

She was referred to an orthopaedic surgeon, but declined surgery, frightened by reports from a friend. Instead she was seen by the occupational therapists who produced a pair of custom built shoes and insoles. They also designed a plastic heel cup to stablize the ankle, but this was soon discarded due to discomfort.

PARTICULAR PROBLEMS IN THE MANAGEMENT OF RHEUMATOID ARTHRITIS

Anaemia

Some degree of anaemia is almost universal in rheumatoid disease. Its cause is usually multifactorial. As some elements are reversible it is always worth reviewing the most likely cause and investigating where necessary.

Anaemia of chronic disease

When the disease is active there is marrow hyperactivity, and often a raised white blood cell and platelet count associated with a moderate normochromic or hypochromic anaemia. This picture is misleading, as the body's iron stores are usually adequate but the normoblasts are unable to make use of the stored iron. Free iron is present in the bone marrow, and the serum iron and iron binding capacity are low. The condition does not improve with oral iron, but only when the disease is suppressed.

Iron-deficiency anaemia

All non-steroidal anti-inflammatory drugs cause irritation of the gastric mucosa and insidious blood loss. Systemic steroids are also associated with bleeding from the gastrointestinal tract. A response to oral iron can be expected if the total iron binding capacity is greater then 55 µmol/l and the serum ferritin level less than 55 µg/l.

Felty's syndrome

This is the association of rheumatoid arthritis with splenomegaly and neutropenia, although often there is a pancytopenia. The cause of this is unknown. Occasionally it will remit naturally. The main danger is the development of agranulocytosis, usually following an infection when the marrow is unable to respond with an adequate leucocytosis. Splenectomy is sometimes useful where there is a persistent pancytopenia, but neither splenectomy nor corticosteroid treatment are reliably effective.

Marrow suppression

Long-acting drugs used in rheumatoid such as gold, D-penicillamine and azathioprine can all cause anaemia as part of marrow suppression. It is for this reason that all patients on these drugs need regular blood counts (usually monthly). There is usually a gradual fall in the white cell or platelet count which reverses as the drug is withdrawn.

Neurological problems

One of the most difficult problems in rheumatoid arthritis is the assessment of an elderly patient with longstanding disability who has 'gone off her legs'. The important question to ask is how much of the locomotor problem is due to painful damaged joints and how much might be due to neurological damage from pressure on the long tracts in the region of the cervical spine. This may present as increasing difficulty with walking, or problems with bladder control. If there is evidence of pressure on the long tracts the patient should be admitted immediately. Surgery to decompress the cervical spine may be necessary to preserve what locomotor power the patient has. The usual cause of this is atlanto-axial subluxation (Fig. 3.7), although there may be subluxation anywhere in the C_2-C_5 segment of the spine.

A number of patients have atlanto-axial subluxation, but no evidence of cord pressure. These patients should be strongly advised to wear a firm collar when travelling and at other times when they are at risk of being jolted or traumatized. Patients with rheumatoid arthritis should be advised never to have manipulative treatment to their necks.

Surgical intervention

Surgery can make a dramatic difference to the functional abilities of a patient with rheumatoid arthritis. The most favourable situation for surgery is when one or two joints are severely affected in the absence of generalized active disease. Replacement arthroplasty at the hip is well

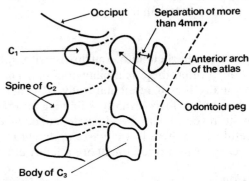

Fig. 3.7. Atlanto-axial subluxation. A lateral X-ray with the neck in flexion shows that separation between the odontoid peg and the arch of the atlas is greater than four millimetres.

established and successful. Excision at the metatarsophalangeal and arthroplasty at the metacarpophalangeal joints gives good pain relief, improves function and, in the former case allows the patient to wear normal shoes. Arthroplasty is less straightforward at the knee and is rarely attempted at the shoulder or elbow. A good review of surgery in rheumatoid arthritis is to be found in Freeman (1986). A summary of common surgical procedures appears in Figure 3.8.

Septic arthritis

This is an occasional complication in a rheumatoid joint. Usually it presents with an acutely tender joint in a toxic patient. Sometimes the onset is insidious, especially in patients on steroids. In general, if a single joint flares up, diagnostic aspiration is essential. If infection is suspected antibiotics should not be given until synovial fluid has been obtained for microbiological examination.

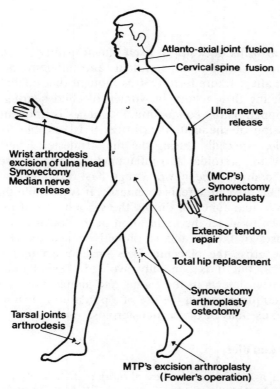

Atlanto-axial joint fusion
Cervical spine fusion
Ulnar nerve release
Wrist arthrodesis
excision of ulna head
Synovectomy
Median nerve
release
(MCP's)
Synovectomy
arthroplasty
Extensor tendon repair
Total hip replacement
Synovectomy
arthroplasty
osteotomy
Tarsal joints
arthrodesis
MTP's excision arthroplasty
(Fowler's operation)

Fig. 3.8. Common surgical procedures in rheumatoid arthritis.

The use of steroids

In the past steroids were used extensively in the treatment of rheumatoid arthritis, with initial dramatic relief of symptoms. However, the long-term complications of steroid treatment are so serious and so frequent (see p. 220) that their use is now reserved for particular problems:

Intolerable pain with progressive disability.
The elderly patient threatened by complete dependency.
Vasculitic complications.
Scleritis.

Local steroid injections can be used more freely. Injection into an inflamed joint, combined with aspiration of any effusion, usually has a transient effect lasting from a few days to several weeks. This may tide a patient over a painful crisis, but is only a temporary solution to an exacerbation in a particular joint. Injection of a mild carpal tunnel syndrome, an inflamed tendon or a tendon nodule, may produce long-lasting relief.

Pregnancy

Rheumatoid arthritis does not in itself affect fertility. As yet there is no clear evidence whether non-steroidal anti-inflammatories, gold or penicillamine affect future fertility. It is thought that penicillamine is the safest slow-acting drug to use in women of child-bearing years, but it should be stopped before conception. Pregnancy is frequently associated with a remission of rheumatoid arthritis. It is sensible to avoid drugs when possible, especially during the first trimester. There is no clear evidence that non-steroidal anti-inflammatory drugs cause early foetal damage, but many of the newer drugs have not been available long enough for their adverse effects to emerge. It is possible that they affect foetal renal vascular function during the second half of pregnancy, and they are known to affect the maturation of the foetal circulation and to delay the onset of labour and so should be avoided. Both gold and penicilliamine cross the placenta; it is unclear whether gold has any adverse effects, but it is generally avoided. Penicillamine can cause connective tissue defects in the foetus and should not be used. During conception and pregnancy, if the use of a potent drug is unavoidable, the safest drugs to use may be the corticosteroids.

Exercise rest and diet

Patients often ask how much they should rest, how much they should exercise, and whether these things damage or help their joints.

Rest

Long periods of bed rest are no longer considered to be a useful form of treatment. Immobilization quickly leads to loss of muscle bulk, and the development of flexion contractures may follow. On the other hand local rest by splinting an acutely inflamed joint will give good pain relief while allowing the patient to regain certain activities. The Occupational Therapy Department will advise on and make up splints.

Daily exercise

This is to be encouraged. Active and resisted exercises build up muscle bulk which protects vulnerable joints. A daily routine of exercises also ensures that joints are put through their maximum range each day, thus preventing the development of contractures. There is increasing evidence that exercise protects against depression and increases a general sense of well-being. There are occasional circumstances when exercise may damage a joint. For example, if there is an unstable valgus or varus deformity at the knee or ankle, repeated weight-bearing exercise will tend to increase the deformity. In this situation a splint to stabilize the joint may be required if surgery is not applicable. The Physiotherapy Department will give useful advice to patients on:

Building up muscle bulk to protect joints.
Prevention of flexion contractures.
Using appliances which minimize the development of deformities.

Diet

At present no clear evidence exists to suggest that particular diets affect the course of the disease, but obese patients put extra stress on their damaged joints and should be encouraged to lose weight.

REFERENCES

Freeman, M. A. R. (1986). Operative surgery in the rheumatic diseases. In Mason and Currey's *Clinical Rheumatology* (4th edn). Currey, H. L. F. (ed). Pitman Medical, London.

Gordon, D. A., Stein, J. L., and Broder, I. (1973). The extra-articular manifestations of rheumatoid arthritis. *Am. J. med.* **54**, 445–52.

Lawrence, J. S. (1977). *Rheumatism in Populations.* Heinemann, London.

Williams, R. C. (ed) (1986). Immunological aspects of rheumatic diseases. *Clinics in Rheumatic Diseases.* **11**, (3) W. B. Saunders, London.

Wright, V. (1986). Regular review: Treatment of severe rheumatoid arthritis. *Br. med. J.* **292**, 431–2.

Zvaifler, N. (1983). Pathogenesis of the joint disease of rheumatoid arthritis. *Am. J. med.* **75**, 3–8.

4 Inflammatory joint disease II:

Other forms of polyarthritis

The classification of inflammatory polyarthritis is untidy and confusing. Until the causes and inter-relationships of these conditions are unravelled it will be necessary to use the type of classification shown in Table 4.1.

Table 4.1. *Classification of inflammatory polyarthritis*

Rheumatoid arthritis	Common at all ages. Usually seropositive. Seronegative cases may represent separate group. Subcutaneous nodules diagnostic.	
Seronegative polyarthritis (spondarthritis)	Ankylosing spondylitis	Usually HLA-B27 positive
	Reiter's disease (a) sexually-acquired (b) dysenteric	
	(Reactive arthritis?)	
	Psoriatic arthritis	Spinal involvement particularly if HLA-B27 positive
	Colitic arthritis	
	(Seronegative rheumatoid arthritis?)	
Juvenile chronic arthritis (Still's disease; JRA)	Systemic type	1–3 years ANA/RF negative
	Polyarticular, rheumatoid factor negative	Younger girls milder
	Polyarticular, rheumatoid factor positive	Older girls resembles adult rheumatoid arthritis
	Oligoarticular Girls < 6 years	Danger of blindness from iritis (especially if ANA positive)
	Oligoarticular Boys > 10 years	HLA-B27 positive: Juvenile onset ankylosing spondylitis

Rheumatoid arthritis (described in Chapter 3) is much the most common and important form of inflammatory polyarthritis. At one time all the disorders mentioned were regarded as varieties of rheumatoid arthritis (e.g. ankylosing spondylitis was 'rheumatoid spondylitis' and childhood polyarthritis was 'juvenile rheumatoid arthritis'). The discovery, in 1948, of the autoantibody rheumatoid factor allowed true rheumatoid arthritis to be separated off from the various seronegative types of polyarthritis. Recently it has become clear that the tissue antigen HLA-B27 is closely linked to the seronegative group of arthropathies, while the disorders in children have been subdivided mainly on the basis of initial clinical presentation.

Despite this classification, all these conditions have features in common. They are systemic disorders, in which synovitis usually affects multiple joints, resulting in the characteristic complaint of early morning stiffness. Affected joints tend to show erosions on X-ray and synovial histological changes are essentially similar. Early in the disease it may be possible only to diagnose inflammatory polyarthritis. The more precise diagnosis of one of the various disorders listed in Table 4.1 will depend on the pattern of joint involvement, any extra-articular clinical features, and the result of laboratory investigations such as tests for rheumatoid factors and HLA-B27.

Generally the 'seronegative' group tends to show more axial (spinal) arthritis, hence the use of the term 'seronegative spondarthritis'. The relationship with HLA-B27 is not understood. This tissue antigen is very closely associated with both ankylosing spondylitis and Reiter's disease. Most patients with psoriatic arthritis do not possess HLA-B27, but those who do are likely to have more spinal involvement, sometimes full blown ankylosing spondylitis. This is an example of the complex overlap between the seronegative arthropathies. Another is the fact that the skin lesions of psoriasis and Reiter's disease are identical, at least histologically. This has led to suggestions that the seronegative arthropathies represent an amorphous group of conditions without clear demarcation, that result from the interplay of predisposing and triggering influences, both genetic (HLA-B27, gender etc) and environmental (infections, inflammatory bowel disease etc) (Brewerton 1985). In practice, the separate labels used in Table 4.1 remain useful for purposes of prognosis and management.

'Seronegative rheumatoid arthritis' remains a difficult diagnostic category. At present it is generally regarded as a benign subgroup of rheumatoid arthritis (see Chapter 3). However, with the passage of time some of these cases evolve into another of the 'seronegative' group (e.g. psoriatic arthritis or ankylosing spondylitis). At a practical level most of these cases behave like (and are managed as) somewhat benign examples of rheumatoid arthritis.

As a group the seronegative arthropathies are less common than rheumatoid arthritis. While the incidence of rheumatoid arthritis is about 2 per cent, ankylosing spondylitis affects about 0.1 per cent of the British population, and both Reiter's disease and psoriatic arthritis are perhaps five times less frequent.

The various conditions listed in Table 4.1 are discussed below (except for rheumatoid arthritis, which is described in Chapter 3).

ANKYLOSING SPONDYLITIS

This form of inflammatory arthritis primarily affects young adult males, and the pattern of joint involvement is centripetal, involving mainly the spine. In severe cases there is a tendency to bony ankylosis. Ninety per cent of patients possess HLA-B27 (compared with 7 per cent in most white populations).

Aetiology

The close link with HLA-B27 points to a strong genetic factor, but how this operates is not understood. Speculation centres round two possibilities: first, that susceptibility depends on a related gene on chromosome 6, perhaps one that determines a particular state of immune reactivity. The second view is that the actual B27 gene product on the cell surface so closely resembles some microbial agent(s) ('molecular mimicry') that exposure to the organisms in question leads to an immune response which cross-reacts with, and damages, host tissues. Alternatively, an organism resembling host tissues may be protected from immune elimination. Aetiological theories have to take account too of the observation that ankylosing spondylitis may sometimes evolve from what starts as typical Reiter's disease, in which 'triggering' of polyarthritis by a transient microbial infection is clearly established. The interplay of genetic, immunological and infective factors which must underlie ankylosing spondylitis is proving surprisingly difficult to unravel.

Epidemiology

About 0.15 per cent of white populations suffer from ankylosing spondylitis. Worldwide the prevalence mirrors the frequency of HLA-B27. It is thus rare in pure blacks, who lack B27. The typical disease affects men five times more frequently than women, and usually starts between the ages of 15 and 25 years. However, tissue typing has revealed that people with B27 may have minor manifestations short of the full blown disease. This includes women, and it may well be that sex determines severity rather than prevalence.

Associated conditions

A variety of disorders occur in association with ankylosing spondylitis. These include peripheral (limb) arthritis (35 per cent), acute anterior uveitis (iritis) (30 per cent), psoriasis (5 per cent), inflammatory bowel disease (ulcerative colitis or Crohn's disease) (5 per cent), cardiac abnormalities (aortic incompetence or conduction defects) (3 per cent). Curiously, the circumstances of the association of these disorders with ankylosing spondylitis suggests that they are neither 'complications' of the disease, nor are they 'triggering' factors which set off the disease. Rather it is as if they are independent conditions to which the individual is susceptible, presumably on a genetic basis.

Clinical features

The presenting complaints in ankylosing spondylitis are often less clearly articular than in the other types of inflammatory arthropathy. A young man will describe rather vague trunk and buttock aches, often of such gradual onset that he has come to regard them almost as 'normal', and the quality of his work or studies may suffer, without anyone being aware that there is a medical explanation. The clue to the correct diagnosis is often the complaint of early morning stiffness, sometimes lasting for hours, or possibly marked relief on taking a non-steroidal anti-inflammatory drug.

The onset may, however, be more dramatic, with acute low backache, sometimes triggered by trauma, and with pain radiating down one leg in a manner mimicking an acute lumbar disc protrusion. Other cases may present with peripheral joint arthritis affecting one or a few lower limb joints. Occasionally inflammatory bowel disease or an attack of iritis may antedate the spondylitis.

In the typical case with gradual onset, the clinical picture suggests early involvement of the sacro-iliac joints, with subsequent spread upwards to involve progressively the lumbar, thoracic and cervical spines. In the most severe cases bony ankylosis spreads to produce a rigid 'poker' spine. Fortunately the disabling forward flexion (kyphotic) deformities which used to accompany this rigidity are preventable by modern management methods. Thoracic spine involvement leads to immobility of the rib cage, so that respiratory movements may become entirely abdominal. Surprisingly this rarely produces any respiratory problems.

Most cases of ankylosing spondylitis are mild and seldom progress to complete spinal ankylosis. For the 30 per cent who develop peripheral arthritis, however, function may be severely impaired (e.g. as in the combination of arthritis of the hip joint with spinal rigidity).

In the non-synovial spinal joints the important factor appears to be inflammation at the junction of tendons and ligaments with bone. Similar 'entheses' may account for pain and tenderness over bony prominences away from joints. The most characteristic is pain in the heel. This may be on the plantar surface (plantar fasciitis) or posteriorly (Achilles' tendinitis). Similar lesions may occur as a feature of Reiter's disease. Other sites, such as the ischial tuberosities may be involved. A painful heel may be an important clue to a B-27-related disease. Such lesions often differ from the more common and familiar forms of painful heel in showing a local, fluffy, periosteal reaction on X-ray.

Early in the course of ankylosing spondylitis, physical examination is likely to reveal one or more of the following tell-tale signs:

1. Irritability of the sacro-iliac joints.
2. Limitation of lumbar spine movement.
3. Restriction of chest expansion.

Irritability of the sacro-iliac joints is revealed by tenderness on firm pressure of the examiner's thumbs over these joints, the surface markings of which are the two dimples best seen by tangential light (Fig. 4.1), and

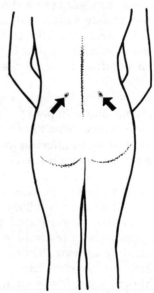

Fig. 4.1. Surface markings of the sacro-iliac joints. The two dimples marking the position of the joints are usually clearly seen with oblique lighting.

also by pain induced in one or both joints when the examiner exerts firm pressure over the centre of the sacrum with the patient lying prone (Fig. 4.2). This manoeuvre produces a slight rotation of the sacrum at the sacro-iliac joints. Lumbar spine flexion is assessed by getting the patient (adequately stripped) to, 'Touch your toes keeping your knees straight'. The examiner views from the side, and the movement is assessed by the change in shape of the lumbar spine, not by the distance the fingers reach. Similarly, lateral bending is assessed by the examiner observing from behind: 'Slide the palm of your left/right hand down the side of your thigh so that you bend sideways without bending forwards'. Ankylosing spondylitis produces restriction of both these movements, whereas lumbar disc lesions tend to produce limitation of flexion while leaving lateral bending intact. Chest expansion is measured with the tape measure at about the level of the male nipple. It should be at least 5 cm.

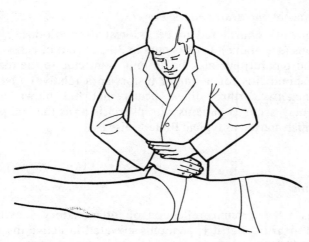

Fig. 4.2. Testing for sacro-iliac irritability. With the patient lying prone the examiner places the ulnar border of the left hand in the upper part of the natal cleft and exerts sharp downward pressure on this with the right hand. A positive test produces pain in one or both sacro-iliac joints.

Complications

Pulmonary problems

These are less common than might be expected in a disease which restricts thoracic breathing. However, a rare form of *apical fibrosis* may mimic tuberculosis.

Spinal fractures

A particular hazard since spinal osteoporosis is combined with rigidity. Selection of recreational activities should take account of this, and headrests are needed in cars.

Amyloidosis

A rare complication.

Romanus lesions

These may occur at the edge of one or more vertebrae, adjacent to the disc. They represent local foci of inflammation and are often painful. On X-ray they appear as bony defects which may closely mimic an infective or neoplastic lesion. They are rare.

Painful heels

Pain in the heels and over other bony prominences is mentioned above.

Lesions of the eye, the heart and the bowel

These lesions are considered to be associated conditions, rather than complications (see above). Iritis occurs in 30 per cent of cases. A history of a red (and painful) eye may be an important clue to the diagnosis of ankylosing spondylitis (or a similar history in a relative). Overlap with other seronegative arthropathies means that full blown ankylosing spondylitis may occur in patients with psoriasis or as the end product of an illness which started as typical Reiter's disease.

Investigations

The ESR is a less reliable reflection of inflammatory activity than in rheumatoid arthritis, but it is generally elevated in active disease. Tests for rheumatoid factor are negative.

X-ray changes are highly characteristic. In the advanced case one can see bony ankylosis between adjacent vertebrae resulting from *syndesmophyte* bridging. These differ from the more horizontal osteophytes of degenerative spondylosis (Fig. 4.3) and, in extreme cases, result in a 'bamboo spine'. Other vertebral changes are osteoporosis and squaring of the outline of the bodies of lumbar vertebrae. The posterior (facetal) joints may also fuse. The fluffy, periosteal, new bone formation over bony prominences has been mentioned above. These changes are late, and do not assist in the diagnosis of the early and mild case. Earlier cases, however, generally show signs of sacro-iliitis on X-ray. These signs comprise irregularity, sclerosis, and erosions, and are usually most

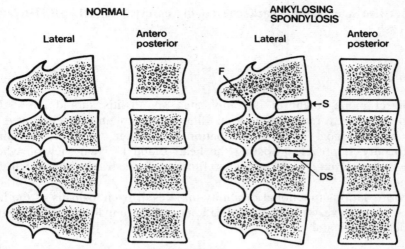

NORMAL

Lateral   Antero posterior

ANKYLOSING SPONDYLOSIS

Lateral   Antero posterior

Fig. 4.3. Radiological changes in ankylosing spondylitis. Vertical syndesmophytes (S) extend from the edges of the vertebrae to give (in advanced cases) the appearance of a 'bamboo spine'. The facetal joints may also fuse (F). In contrast to the appearances in spondylosis (Figure 2.11) note that the syndesmophytes tend to be vertical and the disc spaces (DS) well preserved. In addition, the vertebrae in ankylosing spondylitis tend to be osteoporotic and may show 'squaring' of the contour of the bodies.

obvious on standard views of the pelvis. Later there may be bony fusion. Unfortunately, sacro-iliac changes cannot be reliably identified in subjects below the age of 18 years.

Diagnosis

The full blown picture is unmistakable. However, in the early case the arthritic nature of the pain may be much less clear than in arthropathies involving limb joints. Important clues are a complaint of early morning stiffness, or perhaps a history of episodes of red, painful eyes, or of painful heels (or of these features in a relative). This should lead to a careful assessment of lumbar spine movement, and of chest expansion. The diagnosis can usually be confirmed by the radiological signs of sacro-iliitis, although very rarely these may be absent initially.

About 90 per cent of patients possess HLA-B27 but, testing for this antigen is of limited diagnostic value; in addition, it is an expensive test and is in short supply. The test is unnecessary in the typical case and, because 7 per cent of the normal population are positive, it is unsuitable for screening. It may occasionally be of value in indicating whether an otherwise unexplained backache could represent an HLA-B27-related disease.

Prognosis

Correct management of uncomplicated spondylitis should allow the patient to live a reasonably normal life and to remain fully employed in all but the most physical occupations. A 'poker spine' is a striking deformity. It prevents twisting the head round for rear viewing when driving a car, but it is generally less functionally restrictive than might be expected.

More serious functional disability may result from arthritis of the hip or knee and, very rarely, complications such as amyloidosis or carditis which may be fatal.

Management

Ankylosing spondylitis is a satisfying condition to treat. Spinal symptoms can be controlled by a combination of an anti-inflammatory drug and regular physical exercise. This treatment does not, however, halt progression of the spinal ankylosis, and management of peripheral joint arthritis can be difficult.

Most of the non-steroidal anti-inflammatory drugs have proved effective in treating ankylosing spondylitis. (Phenylbutazone is the most potent but, because of the slight risk of marrow suppression, it is used only when safer drugs are ineffective.) It takes up to one week of medication with these drugs to achieve a full anti-inflammatory effect. They have, therefore, to be taken regularly, rather than 'as required'. The drug chosen should be started at full dosage (e.g. indomethacin 50 mg b.d.) and, once a full effect is obtained, titrated down to the smallest dose which provides adequate symptomatic relief. Trial-and-error may be needed to find the drug which best suits the individual.

Active physical exercise is as important as drug treatment. In order to obtain compliance it is important to prescribe a form of exercise which is actually enjoyed by the patient. Some like a routine of physical jerks; most prefer something more sporting, like swimming or cycling. The essential point is that it must be a regular daily routine or something which demands significant general muscular activity. Ankylosing spondylitis is one disease in which rest is positively harmful. Confinement to bed for some other illness or operation can have a rapidly disasterous effect on mobility and posture unless active physiotherapy is prescribed to prevent it.

It is not understood why physical exercises are so remarkably effective. However, it seems sensible to include a routine of breathing exercises and spinal extension in the hope of minimizing postural deformity.

Most cases should be managed by the GP, with specialist referrals only for particular problems or occasional review. Any progress in spinal deformity should be monitored by recording chest expansion, wall-to-occiput distance (with heels against the wall) and finger-floor distance (bending forwards with knees straight).

X-ray therapy to the spine produces the same symptomatic relief as anti-inflammatory drugs. At one time it was widely used. It has, however, gone out of favour since it increases the risk of myeloid leukaemia by a factor of ten. Radiation is still occasionally used, in doses of up to 1,500 cGy, for those who cannot tolerate anti-inflammatory drugs. It is ineffective for peripheral joint arthritis.

Arthritis of peripheral joints is treated in the same way as rheumatoid arthritis (i.e. with non-steroidal anti-inflammatories), except that slow-acting drugs and systemic corticosteroids are avoided. Surgical replacement of hip joints poses particular problems because, with younger patients, the prosthesis is likely to fail with time, and the tendency to bony overgrowth may shorten the effective functioning of the prosthesis.

Patients require advice about avoiding spinal trauma (because the spine is porotic), and they should be warned about the need for prompt treatment of attacks of iritis (topical mydriatic and corticosteroid drops).

REITER'S DISEASE

Aetiology

Reiter's disease follows either non-specific urethritis or bacillary dysentery, particularly in subjects who possess HLA-B27, and is then, apparently, self-perpetuating. It thus appears to be an immunologically mediated disease, triggered by a microbial infection, and occurring in a genetically-predisposed individual. This concept of a local infection setting off a widespread, non-infective inflammatory disease is the same as that which is thought to operate in 'reactive arthritis', and there is a case for regarding Reiter's disease as 'sexually-acquired reactive arthritis'.

Epidemiology

Reiter's disease is infrequently encountered in general practice, perhaps one case being seen for every five cases of ankylosing spondylitis. Men are affected more than women (20:1) and almost all possess HLA-B27.

The disease usually presents in young adult men, but it is occasionally seen in teenage boys. In British hospitals it is probably diagnosed somewhat more often that psoriatic arthritis. Among males contracting non-specific urethritis, those possessing HLA-B27 have 40 times the risk of developing Reiter's disease. The sexual form is the one usually encountered in Britain. In North Africa and the Middle East the dysenteric form is probably more common.

Clinical features

The patient with the sexually-acquired form of Reiter's disease usually presents with mild, non-specific urethritis within two weeks of sexual intercourse. The urethritis may be so mild as to pass unnoticed, or occasionally there may be an acute haemorrhagic cystitis. Microbiological investigation reveals either *Chlamydia trachomatis* or *Mycoplasma* species in some cases, but not all, and simultaneously acquired gonorrhoea may confuse the issue. Even in the absence of symptoms, genitourinary investigation will reveal evidence of both urethritis and prostatitis. The early morning urine may contain tell-tale threads of purulent material. Effective treatment of urethritis by antibiotics does not influence the subsequent course of Reiter's disease.

The dysenteric type of Reiter's disease follows a bowel infection with *Shigella flexner, S. dysenteriae, S. sonnei,* or other related organisms. In other respects it resembles the sexually-acquired form, although it is notable that patients with dysenteric Reiter's disease may develop 'innocent' urethritis as part of the clinical picture.

The traditional 'classical triad' of Reiter's disease refers to the association of urethritis, conjunctivitis and arthritis. Recently it has been appreciated, first, that the range of clinical features is far wider than the 'triad' and, second, that the disease is probably not a clear-cut separate entity, but merges and overlaps with other seronegative spondarthropathies and B27-related conditions.

Arthritis
This tends to be oligoarticular (affecting one or a few joints) and involves mainly the lower limbs. Sacro-iliitis and spondylitis are features in some patients. The synovitis may be so acute as to suggest pyogenic infection, with erythema of the skin overlying the joint. The arthritis tends to settle over weeks or months, but may be followed, months or years later, by recurrent attacks which lead to chronic joint changes. In some these take the form of chronic lower limb deformities, such as clawed toes. In others there may be features of spinal involvement, sometimes gross ankylosing

spondylitis. These latter patients possess HLA-B27. It is not known to what extent recurrent infections 'trigger' these relapses.

Keratoderma blenorrhagica

Keratoderma blenorrhagica is the characteristic skin lesion. It occurs usually on the soles of the feet, but may spread to produce—in extreme cases—widespread exfoliative dermatitis. Individual lesions start as brown macules, then evolve into papules, then pustules. On the soles the final lesion is a circular flap of white, overhanging skin (the 'iris' lesion) which is highly characteristic. Subungual pustulation and scalp lesions may also occur. Other lesions may be identical with psoriasis. On the glans penis in the uncircumcised, moist superficial ulceration (circinate balanitis) is characteristic, while in the circumcised the lesions are dry and crusted.

Mucosal lesions

In the mouth and pharangeal mucosa these consist of painless superficial ulcers.

Tenosynovitis

This may affect the Achilles' tendon in particular.

Conjunctivitis

This occurs in a minority of cases. It is generally mild and transient.

Iritis and cardiovascular lesions

Both types of lesion may occur as in ankylosing spondylitis.

Neurological lesions

Neurological lesions are rare, but peripheral neuropathy, optic neuritis and meningoencephalopathy have all been described.

Investigations

The ESR reflects inflammatory activity. Tests for rheumatoid factor are negative. HLA-B27 is present in most patients, particularly those with features of spondylitis. Histology of the skin lesions shows features typical of cutaneous psoriasis.

Management

Non-specific urethritis is treated with oxytetracycline 250 mg six-hourly for fourteen days. Treatment of the arthritis is mainly symptomatic, involving non-steroidal anti-inflammatory drugs. Late deformities may require surgical correction. When the arthritis takes the form of ankylosing spondylitis, then the management is as for that disorder. Very rarely, severe systemic involvement may require the administration of corticosteroids. All patients suspected of having sexually-acquired Reiter's syndrome should be seen by a specialist in genitourinary medicine. Exclusion of other sexually-acquired diseases, and an investigation of contacts is necessary.

REACTIVE ARTHRITIS

The concept of a localized bacterial infection 'triggering' a widespread (non-infective) polyarthritis, which then persists or progresses independently of the original infection, is not new. It dates back to early studies into rheumatic fever in which streptococcal pharyngitis acts as the trigger. Recent interest in this idea has been revived by reports that episodes of bacterial infection, particularly bowel infection by Yersinia enterocolitica, may be followed by a self-limiting episode of polyarthritis. A high proportion of these patients possess HLA-B27. In addition, amongst these patients the arthritis tends to be more severe and to involve the spine.

This condition—now referred to as 'reactive arthritis'—is classified with the seronegative spondarthropathies. Clearly, both rheumatic fever and Reiter's disease can be regarded as examples of reactive arthritis, but their well established names are unlikely to be changed at this stage. Some viral arthropathies such as rubella could also be regarded as 'reactive'. However, at present this term is generally reserved for arthropathies which follow defined bacterial infections of the bowel, and which do not have the extra-articular features characteristic of Reiter's disease.

Reactive arthritis is uncommon in Britain. The responsible organisms are usually Yersinia enterocolitica, Salmonella, or Campylobacter. The sexes are equally affected and the arthritis usually appears about one to two weeks after symptoms of dysentery, which may range from very mild to severe. The arthritis may affect one or a few jonts, mainly lower limb, or may occasionally mimic the onset of rheumatoid arthritis. Arthritis generally persists for a few weeks or months, but may be followed by recurrent episodes. Infrequently (and only in patients who possess HLA-B27) the condition may evolve into ankylosing spondylitis. Unless this happens, chronic joint deformities are uncommon.

At a practical level it is important to think of reactive arthritis in those with a recent onset of otherwise unexplained arthritis. An episode of diarrhoea a week or two before the onset may provide the essential clue. Such patients typically possess HLA-B27 but not rheumatoid factor. The 'triggering' organism may be identified either by culture or by a rise and fall in antibody levels. These investigations are best planned in conjunction with the microbiology laboratory.

Any persisting bowel infection may require treatment in its own right, but this will not influence the arthritis. Treatment of the joints is symptomatic.

PSORIATIC ARTHRITIS

One per cent of white populations have the skin condition psoriasis. Of these, about 10 per cent suffer from a seronegative inflammatory polyarthritis. Clinically this may resemble rheumatoid arthritis, but the pattern of joint involvement is often more 'spondylitic' or asymmetrical. Apart from the skin disease and nail involvement, extra-articular features are rare.

Aetiology

Psoriatic arthritis clearly falls within the 'seronegative spondarthritis' group of disorders. As discussed above, there is histological overlap with the cutaneous lesions of Reiter's disease, clinical overlap with ankylosing spondylitis, and a link with HLA-B27. How to interpret this in terms of aetiology is unclear. There is no good evidence of a role for microbial infection, and less evidence for an immunological disturbance than in most of the other inflammatory arthropathies. Women are affected slightly more often than men.

Clinical features

When present, the clinical hallmarks of psoriatic arthritis are highly characteristic. The best known (although relatively uncommon) is inflammatory swelling of the terminal interphalangeal joints of the fingers, with psoriatic deformities of the adjacent nails. The nail lesions may take the form of 'pitting' or other types of deformity such as the 'ladder pattern' (transverse ridging) or subungual hyperkeratosis with nail separation. The terminal interphalangeal joint swelling has to be differentiated from Heberden's nodes and gouty tophi.

Other features suggestive of psoriatic arthritis include:

– Asymmetrical pattern of joint involvement.
– Acute 'explosive' episodes in single finger joints leading to destructive changes.
– Involvement of interphalangeal toe joints.

- (Rare) Widespread severe osteolytic damage to bone ends leading to shortened 'telescoping' digits ('arthritis mutilans').
- Tenosynovitis; in fingers producing 'sausage digits'.
- Any degree of sacroiliitis/spondylitis up to and including full blown ankylosing spondylitis.

One or more of these features in a patient with a seronegative poly-arthritis plus cutaneous psoriasis is accepted as the basis for diagnosing psoriatic arthritis.

Because cutaneous psoriasis and rheumatoid arthritis are both common conditions, they sometimes co-exist in the same patient. When the rheumatoid is seropositive, and nodular, there is no diagnostic difficulty. However, the picture of 'seronegative rheumatoid arthritis' in someone with psoriasis cannot at present be confidently ascribed to either diagnostic category.

Occasionally the polyarthritis appears before the skin changes. If the pattern of joint involvement is sufficiently characteristic, this may allow a diagnosis of probable psoriatic arthritis to be made in the absence of skin lesions.

Apart from the skin changes, extra-articular manifestations of psoriatic arthritis are very rare. Iritis has been described. Amyloidosis is an unusual complication.

The progress of the arthritis is more episodic and asymmetrical than in rheumatoid. Local acute 'explosions' in a single finger joint may lead to severe destructive changes (osteolysis) or to bony ankylosis. Rarely, recurrent episodes of this type may lead eventually to 'arthritis mutilans' with widespread flail, shortened digits and gross disability. In most instances, however, the progress of the arthritis tends to produce less disability than rheumatoid. In general the progress of the arthritis is independent of the fluctuations in the skin disease, although occasionally the skin and the joints may flare simultaneously.

Investigations

As in rheumatoid arthritis, the sedimentation rate and anaemia reflect inflammatory activity. Tests for rheumatoid factor and other autoantibodies are typically negative. HLA-B27 is present in a majority of those who show evidence of spondylitis but usually absent from those who do not. A laboratory curiosity is the fact that cutaneous psoriasis tends to be associated with hyperuricaemia. This can lead to diagnostic confusion with gout. X-ray changes are generally similar to those seen in rheumatoid arthritis, but reflect the somewhat different pattern of joint involvement, including spondylitis in some, and occasionally osteolysis or ankylosis.

Diagnosis

The characteristic features of the arthritis are discussed above. Psoriasis can be unobtrusive and difficult to detect. Careful inspection of the scalp, nails, all the flexures, genitalia and umbilicus is needed to exclude it.

Management

In general the treatment is very similar to that for rheumatoid arthritis except that antimalarial drugs are avoided, as they are thought to exacerbate the skin lesions. Corticosteroids are considered even less desirable than in rheumatoid arthritis, as their withdrawal may precipitate a flare in the skin. Gold is used as a second-line measure and, for exceptionally severe cases, antiproliferative drugs such as methotrexate (particularly for the skin) or azathioprine (particularly for the arthritis) may be tried. Most mild cases can be managed by the GP with non-steroidal anti-inflammatory drugs.

ENTEROPATHIC ARTHRITIS

Patients who suffer from inflammatory bowel disease (ulcerative colitis or Crohn's disease) are liable to develop one of two types of polyarthritis. One is ankylosing spondylitis. As discussed above, this appears to be the association of two separate diseases in a subject who has an independent predisposition to both. These patients generally possess HLA-B27, and the clinical features do not differ from ankylosing spondylitis without bowel disease. The activity of the two diseases waxes and wanes independently, and effective treatment of the bowel disease does not influence the spondylitis.

The other type of polyarthritis is the one to which the name 'enteropathic arthritis' applies. This rare condition is usually a mild oligoarthritis, affecting one or a few, mainly lower limb joints. It behaves like a complication of the bowel disease, appearing after the latter is established, and varying in intensity with the gut inflammation. Further, correcting the bowel problem (by surgery or drugs) is likely to lead to a remission of the arthritis. These patients are seronegative and generally do not possess HLA-B27.

The pathogenesis of this arthritis is unknown. There could be a relationship between it and the somewhat similar oligoarthritis which occurs with erythema nodosum (to which these colitic patients are also liable) or with the arthritis which may complicate therapeutic operations undertaken for obesity.

Usually, symptomatic treatment with non-steroidal anti-inflammatory drugs, physiotherapy, and, perhaps, corticosteroid injections is all that is needed. Very rarely the arthritis is sufficiently severe to become a factor in planning management of the bowel disease.

JUVENILE CHRONIC ARTHRITIS ('STILL'S DISEASE'; 'JUVENILE RHEUMATOID ARTHRITIS')

Inflammatory polyarthritis is fortunately rare in childhood. At one time the general term 'Still's disease' was used to describe all polyarthritis in children under the age of 16 years, and these patients were regarded as having a juvenile form of rheumatoid arthritis. It is now clear that there is a range of such conditions, and they are classified according to the pattern of joint involvement at presentation, and the results of certain laboratory tests (see Table 4.1). These groupings carry important implications for prognosis and management.

Clinical types

Systemic
Young children, usually aged 1–3 years, generally present with systemic features such as fever, rash, lymphadenopathy, hepatosplenomegaly, pericarditis, and pleurisy. Arthritis may not appear until weeks or months after the onset. About one quarter progress to destructive poly-arthritis, the remainder improve after a period of months or years. Tests for rheumatoid factor and anti-nuclear antibody are negative.

Polyarticular, rheumatoid factor negative
This most commonly affects young girls. Systemic features are mild. Ten per cent progress to serious joint destruction.

Polyarticular, rheumatoid factor positive
This type tends to affect older girls and often comes to resemble adult rheumatoid arthritis. Anti-nuclear antibodies are detected in 75 per cent.

Pauci-articular (Oligo-articular)
There are two subgroups of children who present with arthritis of only a few joints (six or less):
   (a) Girls under the age of five. Arthritis is usually mild, but chronic iridocyclitis occurs in 50 per cent, particularly those with positive tests for anti-nuclear antibody. This is insidious (unlike acute iritis in ankylosing spondylitis which is dramatic and unlikely to be missed) and

may lead to blindness. Regular (three to six monthly) ophthalmological screening is therefore mandatory. Rheumatoid factor tests are usually negative.

(b) Older boys. This presents as arthritis of lower-limb-joints but then often progresses into ankylosing spondylitis. A majority possess HLA-B27.

Other types

Occasionally there may be a childhood presentation of psoriatic arthritis, enteropathic arthritis, Reiter's disease, or one of the systemic connective tissue diseases.

Clinical features

In young children it may be difficult to detect arthritis. The relatively greater thickness of articular cartilage means that erosions develop late. Active arthritis can lead to abnormal lengthening or shortening of related long bones such as the metacarpals or metatarsals, or hypoplasia of the mandible may produce a characteristically receding chin. Bony ankylosis, particularly of the neck or wrist, is more common than in the adult. General stunting of growth may occur. A significant proportion of these children develop fatal complicating amyloid disease.

Investigations

The ESR and anaemia reflect disease activity. A neutrophil leucocytosis is usual. Rheumatoid factor and anti-nuclear antibody tests are mentioned above. X-rays differ from those in adult rheumatoid arthritis in showing later appearance of erosions, more periosteal new bone formation, and ankylosis, and sometimes altered length of long bones.

Management

All cases of juvenile chronic arthritis should be seen by a specialist, because of the importance of accurate diagnosis, and deciding a management strategy. Severe cases require management in units experienced in coping with the complex problems of attending to psychological and educational development during a chronic, painful, inflammatory disease. Rest, splinting, physiotherapy, and drugs (broadly similar to those used in adult rheumatoid disease) are the basis of management. Corticosteroids may be required for either joint or extra-articular problems, but carry the risk of stunting growth. Surgery is complicated by the fact that the bones are growing.

REFERENCES

Ansell, B. M. (1980). *Rheumatic Diseases in Childhood*. Butterworth, London.

Craft, A. W. (1985). Arthritis in children. *Br. J. Hosp. Med.* **33**, 188–94.

Craft, A. W. (1985). Management of chronic arthritis in children. *Prescribers' J.* **25**, 75–80.

Fisk, P. (1982). Reiter's disease. *Br. med. J.* **284**, 3–4.

Keat, A. (1983). Reiter's syndrome and reactive arthritis in perspective. *N. Engl. J. Med.* **309**, 1606–15.

Moll, J. M. H. (ed) (1980). *Ankylosing Spondylitis*. Churchill Livingstone, Edinburgh.

Panayi, G. (ed) (1985). Seronegative spondyloarthropathies. *Clinics in Rheumatic Diseases.* **11**(1). W. B. Saunders, London.

Roberts, M. E. T., Wright, V., Hill, A. G. S., and Mehra, C. (1976). Psoriatic arthritis: Follow-up study. *Ann. Rheum. Dis.* **35**, 206–12.

5 Crystal deposition diseases

Gout; pyrophosphate arthropathy

There are three conditions in which metabolic products are deposited in the joints and articular tissues:

1. Gout, in which urate crystals are deposited in the small peripheral joints.
2. Pyrophosphate arthropathy (pseudogout, chondrocalcinosis), in which calcium pyrophosphate is deposited in the cartilage of the larger limb-joints.
3. Ochronosis, a very rare condition in which homogentisic acid is deposited in the cartilage of the central (spinal) joints.

GOUT

Gout is the peripheral arthropathy resulting from sustained hyper-uricaemia. It is the commonest hazard associated with a high circulating concentration of urate.

Incidence

In 1975 a study by W. J. Currie looked at the epidemiology of gout in 64 general practices throughout Britain. The prevalence was found to be 2.6/1000 population, with a male:female ratio of 6:1. The section of the population most at risk was men over 45 years of age, of whom 1 per cent were found to have symptomatic gout. Table 5.1 demonstrates the regional variation in prevalence.

The majority of cases in this study were classified as primary gout. Only 10 per cent were thought to be secondary, and among this small group diuretic therapy was by far the most common causal agent. Other studies suggest that asymptomatic hyperuricaemia is about ten times as

Table 5.1. *The regional variation in the prevalance of gout*

Region	Incidence/1000 in 1975	Prevalence in 1975
Scotland	0.17	1.3
Wales	0.17	2.1
England	0.35	3.0

common as gout, and once again the commonest cause is the use of diuretics.

Urate metabolism

Urate is the end product of purine metabolism. The plasma urate concentration is determined mainly by the rate of purine metabolism and the rate of urate excretion by the kidney. Both these factors are determined, in part, by genetic factors, but can also be modified by disease, drugs and diet.

The renal handling of urate is complex. In brief, urate appears in the glomerular filtrate, is largely reabsorbed in the proximal tubule, and actively secreted more distally. A number of drugs and metabolic products interfere with the active transport of urate within the kidney, hence disturbing the plasma urate concentration. Figure 5.1 summarizes the factors affecting the plasma urate concentration; a good review of this complex subject can be found in Boss and Seegmiller (1979).

For practical purposes hyperuricaemia is divided into:

1. Primary in which there may be a genetically-based increase in urate synthesis (over producers), or a reduction in the rate of renal excretion (under excretors). This accounts for the majority of cases.
2. Secondary in which the hyperuricaemia has an acquired cause. The commoner causes include:
   (a) Increased purine turnover as a result of myeloproliferative disorders, other neoplasms, severe psoriasis.
   (b) Decreased renal excretion as a result of renal disease, endocrine disease (myxoedema, hyperparathyroidism), acidosis, alcohol,

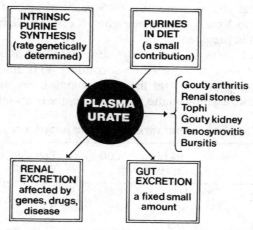

Fig. 5.1. Factors affecting the plasma urate concentration.

starvation, exercise, or drugs (e.g. thiazides, low-dose aspirin, ethambutol).

Pathogenesis

During an acute attack of gout, urate crystals form within the joint cavity. This triggers the inflammatory response. The crystals are phagocytosed by leucocytes which rupture to release lysozymes and other chemical mediators of inflammation. In chronic gout, deposits of urate settle in the articular structures, destroying the surface of the cartilage and the under-lying bone and stimulating changes similar to those found in osteo-arthritis. Urate deposits (tophi) can also appear in other cartilaginous structures such as the helix of the ear—where tophi should always be sought (Fig. 5.2)—and within bursae and tendons.

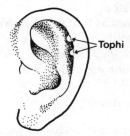

Fig. 5.2. Tophi in the helix of the ear.

Clinical presentation

Podagra, acute gout of the first metatarsophalangeal joint, is the most common presentation of gouty arthritis. The pain develops rapidly and within a few hours the joint is swollen and exquisitely tender, the over-lying skin being hot and red. Usually the patient cannot bear anything to touch the joint; occasionally he will be generally unwell and feverish. Untreated, the acute attack settles over a week or two leaving the joint perfectly normal.

This classic presentation should not blind one to the diverse manifesta-tions of gout. Acute gout may present as an acutely painful synovitis in any small joint, and less frequently in a larger joint such as the knee or elbow. The pain, surrounding inflammation and systemic upset may mimic a septic arthritis or cellulitis. On the other hand gout may also produce quite a mild bout of synovitis, and repeated mild attacks may be mis-diagnosed as trauma or osteoarthritis if they settle before the patient is seen. Usually only one joint is involved at a time, but a small proportion of patients have polyarticular attacks.

Some patients may experience only one or two attacks of gout in their lifetime. However, those with the largest pool of accumulated urate will, if untreated, progress over several years to chronic tophaceous gout. In this severe form of the disease, repeated attacks of acute gout, in association with urate deposits in the cartilage and bone, cause progressive joint damage. The picture is then of a grumbling asymmetrical polyarthritis punctuated by acute exacerbations in a few joints.

DIAGNOSIS AND MANAGEMENT

Faced with a single, acutely inflamed joint the following differential diagnoses should be considered:

Trauma
Gout
Sepsis
Pyrophosphate arthropathy
Seronegative arthritis such as Reiter's or psoriatic arthritis
Monoarticular rheumatoid
Palindromic rheumatism (p. 31).
Peri-articular inflammation e.g. cellulitis in the foot, prepatellar bursitis

Management of the acute attack

Initial management of the acute attack in general practice often has to precede a firm diagnosis.

Full doses of indomethacin (50 mg t.d.s) or naproxen (250 mg t.d.s.) will reliably cut short an attack, and are the recommended first line of treatment. Phenylbutazone should be avoided because of its potentially serious side-effects. Aspirin should be avoided as it blocks the renal secretion of urate unless used in very high doses which may cause side-effects.

Colchicine, which interferes with leucocyte function, was used extensively in the past; it is slightly less effective than the non-steroidal anti-inflammatory drugs, with more side-effects. It is given as 1 mg stat, followed by 0.5 mg every two or three hours until the symptoms cease or vomiting and diarrhoea supervene.

Aspiration of the joint and local steroid injection is probably the quickest way of aborting an attack. It also provides joint fluid for crystal examination. However, this is not always practicable and the patient may be unwilling to have a joint needled when it is at its most tender.

Diagnosis

The upper limit of the normal range of plasma urate is 440 μmol/l for men and 380 μmol/l for women, although these levels may vary some-what between laboratories. Many individuals with a raised plasma urate are asymptomatic, hence a raised level on its own does not confirm a diagnosis of gout. A typical clinical history in combination with a raised urate level is presumptive evidence of gout, and for all practical purposes a repeatedly normal urate level in the absence of treatment is inconsistent with the diagnosis.

The most conclusive method of diagnosis is by direct observation of urate crystals with a polarizing light microscope (see Appendix 1). Joint fluid or material from a tophus are suitable for this method, no special preservative is needed for the container, and immediate examination is not essential. If necessary the specimen can be posted to a laboratory with the appropriate facilities.

X-rays. Urate is radiolucent, so the diagnosis cannot be made radiologically. In long-standing tophaceous gout the urate deposits may cause punched out erosions in the bone surface, and tophi may become calcified. In addition, the non-specific changes of secondary osteo-arthritis may be present.

Management of chronic gout

Untreated gout shows a wide range of severity. The mildly affected patient may have only one or two bouts of crystal synovitis in a lifetime, while the severely affected patient will have a progressive crippling arthritis with associated renal damage which may prove fatal.

In general there is no indication to start someone on prophylactic medication after a first attack of gout. Instead patients should be given a supply of non-steroidal anti-inflammatory drugs to start as early as possible in the course of an attack, and should be warned about things which may trigger the condition. These include: local trauma; excessive exercise, starvation or alcohol excess — these are causes of metabolic acidosis which decreases the tubular excretion of urate; obesity, the urate concentration falls as weight is lost.

Their drug regimen should be scrutinized, and other causes of secondary gout excluded. Alcohol intake should be restricted to modest amounts, but there is no need to change the average diet, as dietary intake exerts only a modest effect on the urate concentration. It is important to monitor the blood pressure, as there is an increased incidence of hypertension and ischaemic heart disease in gout sufferers. Early evidence of renal involvement should be sought by testing the urine for protein and checking the plasma creatinine.

Prophylactic treatment should be considered if:

1. There are recurrent acute attacks; more than one or two in a year.

2. Tophi are present; this reflects a high total-body urate pool and a poor prognosis.
3. Evidence of renal involvement; either as urate stones, or as 'gouty kidney', which may show itself initially as proteinuria and progress to hypertension and renal insufficiency.
4. In some causes of secondary gout: e.g. the highly cellular neoplasms, especially during treatment. This is to prevent intra-tubular depositon of uric acid crystals leading to acute renal failure.

The first choice for prophylactic treatment is allopurinol. This is an inhibitor of the enzyme xanthine oxidase and hence reduces the production of urate. To date this has proved a safe drug, with very few side-effects; it should be used in a reduced dose in renal failure. The drug is introduced at a dose of 100 mg daily, and increased to a maintenance dose of 200–500 mg so as to maintain the urate concentration within the normal range. In the first month of starting treatment there is an increased risk of precipitating an acute attack of gout, so during this period either a non-steroidal anti-inflammatory drug or colchicine (1 mg daily) should be used as preventive treatment.

If allopurinol cannot be used a uricosuric drug may be tried. These drugs paralyse the renal tubular transport of urate, producing a marked urate diuresis. Probenecid and sulphinpyrazone are equally effective. Both may cause acute attacks during their introduction, and are not suitable for patients prone to stone formation. They are ineffective in the presence of renal failure.

Particular problems in the management of gout

Asymptomatic hyperuricaemia
Clinicians vary in their attitude towards this condition. It is not uncommon for patients with a plasma urate above 600 µmol/l to be started on allopurinol in spite of never having had an attack of gout. It would seem sensible to do this if there is evidence of renal impairment, but in the absence of this it would be reasonable to maintain a watching brief with a regular review of renal function, rather than embark upon lifelong medication.

Gout, hypertension and the kidney
As gout and hypertension are linked conditions, a not uncommon clinical conundrum is presented by a man who has had a single attack of gout, has hypertension, and is found to have proteinuria. Is it the hypertension or the gout? Should he be on allopurinol? There is no clearcut answer to this. Renal function should be reviewed regularly, and prophylactic treatment started if there is evidence of decline.

Minimal renal insufficiency is found in about 50 per cent of gouty patients, but as many of these patients will be suffering from age-related changes it is difficult to be sure about the exact contribution of the hyperuricaemia. Proteinuria, without other signs of renal disorder, is found in about 25 per cent of gouty patients, and in general is mild and not progressive. Chronic urate nephropathy is rare and is associated with severe tophaceous gout of some years standing. Its causes are not well understood, but the kidneys show a combination of glomerulosclerosis, interstitial urate deposits and changes of pyelonephritis. Patients with this condition progress very slowly to chronic renal insufficiency.

Nephrolithiasis in gouty subjects may be caused either by pure uric acid stones which are radiolucent, or mixed uric acid and calcium oxalate stones. They are an indication for treatment with allopurinol. An increased fluid intake and alkalinization of the urine to a pH above 6.0 will decrease the tendency of uric acid crystals to precipitate out.

PYROPHOSPHATE ARTHROPATHY

Pyrophosphate arthropathy (pseudo-gout or chondrocalcinosis) has only recently been distinguished from gout. When polarized light microscopy was used to look for urate crystals in patients with acute arthritis some specimens contained non-urate crystals. In due course these were identified as calcium pyrophosphate dihydrate, and it has now become clear that these are a common cause of joint pathology.

Prevalence

Half of the elderly population who come to post-mortem have evidence of pyrophosphate deposition in their joint cartilage. During life, X-ray evidence of asymptomatic chondrocalcinosis is a common finding in the elderly, particularly in the menisci of the knee. A much smaller group have symptomatic disease.

The condition commonly presents in the sixth or seventh decade of life, and is usually 'primary'. A minority of cases are 'secondary', associated with hypercalcaemia (e.g. in hyperparathyroidism), or haemochromatosis.

Although there is no doubt that pyrophosphate crystals can cause a painful synovitis, there is uncertainty as to whether it is the presence of a damaged joint surface which triggers the crystal deposition, or whether the pyrophosphate crystals are causative in the generation of chronic arthritis. The situation is further confused by the presence of hydroxy-apatite crystals in some osteoarthritic joints. These are too small to be seen with the polarizing light microscope, but there is speculation that their presence may contribute to the acute flares seen in osteoarthritis.

Clinical presentation

Pyrophosphate arthropathy manifests itself in three ways:

Recurrent attacks of acute arthritis (pseudo-gout)
The commonest joint to be affected is the knee, but other large joints—the hips, shoulders and elbows—may also be involved. The acute attack, which is caused by crystals entering the joint space, may mimic gout or even a septic arthritis. The untreated joint will begin to settle after about ten days, but residual synoval inflammation tends to grumble on for several weeks.

Chronic degenerative arthritis
Some patients never experience an acute attack, but develop a progressive, degenerative joint disease clinically very similar to osteoarthritis. This is caused by crystals deposited within the cartilage leading to degenerative changes. Indeed, the combination of generalized osteoarthritis with radiological evidence of chondrocalcinosis is quite common and it is difficult to separate the contribution of each pathology to the patient's condition. Fortunately this is not important for practical management, as current treatment of the two conditions is similar.

Chronic arthritis with episodes of acute synovitis
Commonly a patient who is thought to have osteoarthritis will have several acute exacerbations of joint inflammation, usually affecting the knee. Pyrophosphate deposition will eventually be noticed on an X-ray or when the swollen joint is aspirated. Probably many patients who have mild attacks never have the condition recognized. The contribution of hydroxyapatite crystals to these episodes of synovitis remains speculative (see above).

Diagnosis and management

X-rays of affected joints will show a line of calcification parallel to the bone cortex, lying in the surface of the hyaline cartilage (see Fig. 5.3), in the knee the menisci may also show calcification.

The most useful joint to screen is the knee, followed by the wrist, symphisis pubis and shoulder.

Examination of the synovial fluid during an acute attack will show crystals of pyrophosphate. These exhibit weak positive birefringence when viewed with a polarizing light microscope. As for gout, a plain container is used for collection of the fluid, and the specimen need not be examined immediately.

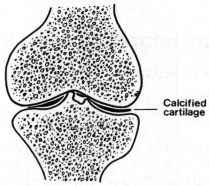

Calcified
cartilage

Fig. 5.3. Chondrocalcinosis in the knee joint. X-rays show a line of calcification in the articular cartilage. It is often seen in the menisci as well.

Investigations

The majority of cases are primary. Hypercalcaemia should be excluded, and haemochromatosis should be remembered as a rare cause.

Treatment

The most effective treatment for the acute attack is aspiration of the joint and injection of a steroid preparation. Unlike gout, in which pain relief from indomethacin occurs rapidly, non-steroidal anti-inflammatory drug medication gives some help, but the attack may still grumble on for a week or so. The management of chronic chondrocalcinosis is similar to that of osteoarthritis.

REFERENCES

Boss, G. R. and Seegmiller, J. E. (1979). Hyperuricaemia and gout: classification, complications and management. *N. Engl. J. Med.* **300**, 1459–67.

Currie, W. J. (1979). Prevalance and incidence of gout in Great Britain. *Ann. Rheum. Dis.* **36**, 101–4.

Nuki, G. (1979). Gout and hyperuricaemia. *Medicine* (3rd series) **14**, 700.

6 Systemic connective tissue diseases

('Collagen Diseases')

INTRODUCTION

A number of rare and often serious diseases are grouped together under the title 'systemic connective tissue diseases' (Table 6.1). They are grouped together because of features which they have in common (Table 6.2) and which suggest that, pathologically, they are closely related.

Much the most important of these is rheumatoid arthritis. It is discussed in Chapter 3. Giant cell arteritis is so closely linked with the important condition *polymyalgia rheumatica* that it is discussed separately in Chapter 7.

The precise diagnostic distinction between these various systemic connective tissue diseases may be difficult, even after intensive investigation, and the management (often unsatisfactory) usually demands collaboration between primary care and specialized hospital departments.

Perhaps the most important responsibility in primary medical care is to recognize that one of these conditions may exist. Apart from rheumatoid

Table 6.1. *Systemic connective tissue diseases*

Systemic lupus erythematosus
Systemic sclerosis (scleroderma)
Polyarteritis nodosa
Dermatomyositis and polymyositis
Mixed connective tissue disease
Sjøgren's syndrome
Rheumatoid arthritis

Table 6.2. *Features common to the systemic connective tissue diseases*

Involvement of multiple systems; usually including vasculitis and arthritis.

'Overlap': patients may present with features of more than one of these disorders or, over a period change from one diagnosis to another.

Evidence of an immunological mechnaism producing the disease; e.g. circulating immune complexes and autoantibodies, and altered immune regulation.

Unknown aetiology.

arthritis, the presenting features are often confusing. Some of the pointers which may alert the clinician to this possibility are shown in Table 6.3.

Once suspicion is aroused, the most useful general screening tests are the ESR and a search for circulating autoantibodies such as anti-nuclear antibodies and rheumatoid factors (latex test). Indications for more detailed investigations are given in the sections below dealing with the individual conditions. The final allocation of a patient to one or other of these disease categories may remain a matter for speculation even after the most intensive investigation. Furthermore, as mentioned above, individual patients may apparently change from one diagnostic category to another. In these circumstances is it important to make a precise diagnosis? The answer must be 'yes', for both prognosis and management strategy depend on the diagnosis.

Table 6.3. *Some clinical features which may alert the clinician to the presence of a systemic connective tissue disease*

Multiple system involvement, e.g. skin, joints, and kidneys

Raynaud's phenomenon, especially when it appears for the first time in an adult

Arthralgia

Characteristic skin lesions such as sclerodactyly, livedo reticularis, butterfly rash, or purpura

Proximal muscle weakness

SYSTEMIC LUPUS ERYTHEMATOSUS (SLE)

This is the most obviously 'autoimmune' of the rheumatic diseases. It affects mainly women of child-bearing age and may involve almost any system in the body. Thus, although rare, its exclusion by appropriate screening tests is necessary in patients with widely differing clinical presentations.

Aetiology and pathogenesis

The best studied lesion is lupus nephritis. This appears to result from the deposition of immune complexes (probably consisting of DNA/anti-DNA) on the glomerular basement membrane. These complexes activate the complement cascade, leading to local inflammation. It seems likely that many of the diverse features of the disease depend on immune complex deposition in vessel walls at different sites. In general there is intense immunological overactivity, and a variety of autoantibodies can be detected in the blood. It appears that the central event is a loss of control of immunological regulation, allowing 'self' antigens to be treated as 'foreign'. The trigger for this disturbance is unknown. It might depend on the interaction of an environmental factor (e.g. a virus) with an inborn host factor (e.g. a particular pattern of immune reactivity).

Clinical features

In Britain one case of SLE is seen for about 20 cases of rheumatoid arthritis and females outnumber males by 10:1. The onset is most often during the child-bearing years. There is slight familial clustering.

SLE tends to follow an episodic, relapsing course, sometimes with long periods of relative inactivity punctuated by acute life-threatening episodes. Such relapses may be precipitated by exposure to sunlight or drugs. Almost any organ may be affected.

Skin lesions

These are the most common feature. They may be triggered by sunlight exposure. The well-known (but uncommon) 'butterfly rash' consists of erythema of the cheeks joined across the bridge of the nose. Purpura and other types of cutaneous vasculitis (p. 85) are common, while the skin at the base of the finger nails may show a characteristic mixture of erythema and telangiectasia associated with pitted scarring of the finger pulps. Other cutaneous features include Raynaud's phenomenon and loss of hair, or there may be overlap with the skin lesions of dermatomyositis or scleroderma. 'Chronic discoid lupus' appears to be a benign, local variant of SLE in which a 'butterfly rash' progresses to chronic scarring and pigmentation. These patients may have circulating anti-nuclear antibodies and occasionally develop mild systemic features.

Joint involvement

This occurs in most patients. It may mimic rheumatoid arthritis with synovitis of many joints, but radiological erosions and destructive changes are rare. Often there is only arthralgia (joint pains without evidence of synovitis). Aseptic necrosis (p. 182) is a rare complication.

Cardiovascular involvement

This may produce chest pain due to pericarditis. Less often myocarditis may lead to heart failure, or endocardial lesions may cause cardiac murmurs (verrucose endocarditis of Libman-Sacks). Peripheral vasculitis is common. The clinical signs depend on the size of the vessel involved, varying from skin purpura to necrotic ulcers or gangrene of a digit.

Respiratory involvement

This most commonly produces pleuritic chest pain, which can be very persistent. Pleural effusions, pulmonary infiltrates and changes in lung function may occur (diffusion defects or 'shrinking lungs').

Renal disease

Is an important cause of death, and established renal disease is a bad prognostic omen. Kidney involvement may be revealed by proteinuria, haematuria, urinary casts, hypertension or impaired renal function. At first these changes are reversible. Once established they are likely to progress either to renal failure with hypertension or to a nephrotic syndrome. There is evidence that renal disease develops and progresses when laboratory tests (see below) reveal high levels of DNA binding and low complement levels (indicating immune-complex formation). These circumstances are therefore regarded as indications for aggressive therapy.

The eye

This may be affected by Sjøgren's syndrome (p. 91), optic neuritis or retinopathy (including the round white exudates known as 'cytoid bodies').

Haematological involvement

Is most often revealed by leucopenia (particularly lymphopenia). This can be a useful diagnostic clue. Other blood changes include auto-immune haemolytic anaemia and thrombocytopenic purpura. Either of these may occur as dramatic life-threatening episodes. The haematological features resemble the 'idiopathic' forms of these conditions. Coagulation tests may reveal the 'lupus anticoagulant'. This rarely causes bleeding problems, but may—paradoxically—be associated with thrombosis (see anti-cardiolipin antibody under Investigations).

Neuropsychiatric involvement

Carries a sinister prognosis. The most common problem is chronic headache, often with migrainous characteristics. Minor psychiatric changes are not uncommon and occasionally a frank psychosis develops. Cerebral arteritis may lead to epilepsy, hemiplegia or cranial nerve palsies. Other neurological features include myelopathy and neuropathy.

Other clinical features

These include splenomegaly, lymphadenopathy, abdominal pain and myopathy.

DRUG-INDUCED SLE

The relationship of drugs and SLE is complex. Sensitivity reactions to many drugs appear capable of triggering relapses in patients with SLE. For this reason drugs (e.g. penicillin) should never be prescribed for these patients unless the indications are absolutely clear. A more specific relationship exists with drugs such as hydrallazine, procainamide, methyldopa and chlorpromazine. Continued administration of these drugs to apparently normal people may cause anti-nuclear antibodies to appear in the circulation, and in some subjects a lupus-like clinical syndrome is produced. Characteristically this is more benign than ordinary SLE in that neurological and renal involvement are rare, the condition remits on withdrawing the drug, and tests for anti-double-stranded DNA ('DNA binding') are negative. However, this is not always the case, and it appears possible that drugs such as hydrallazine may trigger full-blown SLE in a minority of people who are perhaps pre-disposed to the disease, while others develop only the benign syndrome. At one time it was believed that induction of lupus required relatively large doses of hydrallazine, and that low doses were safe. Recent reports indicate that even quite modest doses of the drug may sometimes set off the lupus syndrome.

'Lupoid hepatitis'

Women with chronic, active hepatitis are liable to develop anti-nuclear antibodies (but not positive DNA-binding tests) and features such as arthritis which mimic SLE. By contrast, liver changes are uncommon in SLE. At one time this 'lupoid hepatitis' was regarded as a variant of SLE. It is now considered to be a completely separate disorder.

Laboratory investigations (see also Appendix 1)

The ESR reflects the inflammatory activity of the disease. By contrast, C-reactive protein levels tend to be normal in uncomplicated lupus, and to rise only if there is complicating infection. Active disease is associated with a mild anaemia.

The basis for the diagnosis of SLE is the presence of circulating auto-antibodies directed against nuclear components. There are three standard tests (see also Appendix 1):

1. LE CELL TEST. This is a reasonably reliable test (although somewhat non-specific), but it is too time consuming for routine use.
2. FLUORESCENT ANTI-NUCLEAR ANTIBODY TEST. This simple and cheap test is highly sensitive, but positive results

may be obtained in patients who do not have SLE. It is an excellent screening test for lupus.
3. ANTIBODIES TO NATIVE (DOUBLE-STRANDED) DNA. A radioactive immune assay (DNA-binding test) or a fluorescent test using *Crithidia luciliae* can be used to detect antibodies directed specifically against native (double-stranded) DNA. This is a highly specific test for SLE, but relatively insensitive. Some definite cases give negative results.

Other autoantibodies

The serum of lupus patients may contain a very wide variety of other autoantibodies directed against nuclear or cytoplasmic antigens, or rheumatoid factors. Of recent interest are antibodies to phospholipid. These account for 'lupus anticoagulant' activity as well as 'false positive tests for syphilis'. This antibody rarely causes bleeding problems, but it is associated with thrombotic episodes, abortions and CNS involvement. It is occasionally a pointer to SLE in a patient in whom the anti-nuclear antibody test is negative.

Circulating immune complexes

These can be detected in most cases of active SLE.

Complement levels

These are lowered (through consumption) during periods of immune-complex formation. The combination of falling complement levels and rising DNA-binding values (see above) is thought to herald an active phase of the disease with the threat of renal involvement (and thus may call for more aggressive therapy).

Band test

Fluorescent microscopy of skin obtained by punch biopsy from an exposed (but uninvolved) area may reveal complement and immuno-globulin (markers of immune complexes). This can be a useful pointer to the diagnosis.

Renal biopsy

Apart from excluding other conditions such as amyloidosis, a renal biopsy can indicate the severity of renal lupus. Early proliferative changes are reversible. Crescent formation indicates a poor prognosis.

Diagnosis

Florid lupus is unmistakable. Difficulty arises when a single system is involved. Fortunately the screening tests (ESR plus ANA) are reliable and inexpensive. The important thing is to remember to use them. They should be routine tests in anyone who develops otherwise unexplained arthritis, psychosis, focal neurological lesions, Raynaud's phenomenon or autoimmune haematological disorders. A positive DNA-binding test confirms the diagnosis of SLE. Differentiation from rheumatoid can be difficult (but is important because of differences in treatment and prognosis). There may be positive anti-nuclear antibody and latex tests in both conditions, but the progressive, erosive joint disease of rheumatoid arthritis is rare in SLE.

Management

Patients should be warned to avoid unnecessary sunlight exposure and drugs for which there is not a clear indication.

Corticosteroids are the only drugs which effectively suppress lupus activity, but this may require high dosages. Long-term administration produces so many undesirable side-effects that steroids are if possible reserved for 'fire extinguisher' use. In other words they are employed in short, sharp, courses to tide the patient over serious disease flares (e.g. autoimmune haematological disease, severe vasculitis or advancing renal disease). In these circumstances large doses are given over a limited period, e.g. prednisolone 50–100 mg daily by mouth or methylprednisolone 1 g by intravenous infusion daily for a few days. Between acute flares the drug is stopped or titrated down to the minimum needed to control disease activity.

Immunosuppressive drugs (e.g. cyclophosphamide or azathioprine) appear to augment the suppressive effect of corticosteroids in renal lupus. In other circumstances their value is unproven. They are, however, generally added to the regimen of severe cases of lupus when other drugs fail to control the disease.

Antimalarials have a modestly favourable effect on mild SLE. For example, in patients with skin and joint complaints only, it is worth giving hydroxychloroquine 200 mg daily (with ophthalmological surveillance every three to six months for retinal toxicity).

Joint pains, renal failure, epilepsy, hypertension etc., require management in their own right.

More aggressive methods of suppressing immunity such as plasmapheresis, leucopheresis, anti-lymphocyte globulin, thoracic duct drainage, and total lymphoid irradiation have not yet found a clear role in management.

Prognosis

SLE is a sinister diagnosis to make, and established renal lupus carries a bad prognosis. However, very mild cases (with perhaps just arthralgia or occasional episodes of pericardial or pleural pain) are not uncommon. Most lupus patients require regular medical supervision, and their lives are often distressingly disturbed by the disease. However, survival is better than might be expected, and may be improving. The immediate cause of death is often secondary infection. Perinatal mortality is increased, but pregnancy is not contraindicated unless the patient has progressive renal disease or a psychosis.

SYSTEMIC SCLEROSIS (SCLERODERMA)

Scleroderma describes the main skin manifestation of this rare disease: hardening and tethering of the skin which affects mainly the fingers. A similar process involves internal organs such as the lungs, kidneys, and heart, leading usually to death. The cause is unknown, and it is uncertain whether vascular insufficiency or connective tissue sclerosis is the primary event. There is close overlap with both SLE and polymyositis.

Clinical features

Women are affected three times more often than men and the onset is usually between the ages of 30 and 50 years. The presenting symptom is typically Raynaud's phenomenon, the patient complaining that exposure to cold causes her fingers to turn white and numb. This is due to digital artery spasm. After a period of five to fifteen minutes the fingers take on a mottled appearance (due to capillary dilatation), then finally turn pink again as the arteries dilate. These familiar colour changes are relatively common amongst school girls during cold weather. However, when it appears for the first time in adult life, Raynaud's phenomenon has sinister implications. The closest link is with systemic sclerosis, but it is sometimes the first warning of one of the other connective tissue diseases (Table 6.1).

After weeks or months of Raynaud's phenomenon the patient notices that the skin over the fingers is becoming harder and tethered to under-lying tissues (acrosclerosis). At this stage there is often a mild synovitis of the finger joints which prevents the patient making a tight fist.

Examination of the hands reveals a waxy thickening of the skin of the fingers (sclerodactyly) and slight swelling of the finger joints. In a typical case the sclerosis spreads gradually to involve the forearms, face, and the front of the chest. Very rarely the whole trunk may become hidebound. The transition from normal to abnormal skin is gradual and indistinct (differentiating scleroderma from other conditions such as morphoea in which the edge of the lesion is clearly demarcated). Careful inspection shows other changes in the skin. Telangiectasia is common on the hands and face; irregular patches of both pigmentation and depigmentation appear; skin appendages are lost, giving the skin a shiny, monotonous appearance. Later there is soft tissue calcification producing visible and palpable nodules which show well on X-ray. Loss of subcutaneous tissue produces pointed finger tips (poikiloderma) and ischaemic skin ulceration is common. Tenosynovitis often occurs early. This may limit finger movements and produce palpable crepitus (appreciated by gripping the distal forearm while the patient opens and closes her fist). The face takes on a characteristic appearance with a small mouth opening (microstomia) and creases radiating outwards from the lips.

These visible changes, which may range from subtle finger sclerosis to widespread 'armour plating' of the whole trunk, represent the scleroderma component of this disease. A simultaneous process of collagen sclerosis affects internal organs. Oesophageal hypomotility is common and often appears early. It may be asymptomatic or produce dyspepsia or dysphagia. It is revealed by barium swallow performed in the head-down position. Pulmonary involvement may produce an impairment in gas diffusion, restrictive disease, pleural effusion or pulmonary hypertension. Cardiac problems are common. These are usually secondary to either pulmonary or systemic hypertension, but pericarditis, myocarditis, or aortic valve lesions may also occur. Renal lesions are an important cause of death. Both renal failure and hypertension are serious hazards. The latter may be 'malignant' and rapidly progressive. It appears that corticosteroids may provoke or aggravate hypertension (to a much greater extent than in normal subjects). Involvement of the small intestine may produce malabsorption.

'CREST' syndrome

This term is used to describe the clinical picture in what may possibly be a relatively benign subgroup of patients with systemic sclerosis. The acronym refers to the association of calcinosis, Raynaud's phenomenon, oesophageal involvement, sclerodactyly, and telangiectasis. In the serum, anticentromere autoantibodies are particularly common. Whether this represents a distinct subgroup with a better prognosis is not yet established. The older term Thibiege–Weissenbach syndrome refers to the association of telangiectasia, sclerodactyly, and calcinosis.

Investigations (see also Appendix 1)

The ESR is usually moderately raised, and most patients have circulating autoantibodies. The anti-nuclear antibody test is generally positive, often in a 'speckled' pattern (see Appendix 1). More specific for systemic sclerosis are the anti-centromere and 'Scl 70' antibodies. Rheumatoid factors may also by detected.

Management

No treatment is available which will halt the advance of the more severe case. Prednisolone will relieve the early synovitis, but the danger of precipitating hypertension probably precludes its use. Raynaud's phenomenon is managed by keeping the hands and the body generally warm.

When skin viability is threatened it may be justifiable to undertake cervical sympathectomy or administer prostaglandin E_1 or nifedipine. The blood pressure must be monitored and any hypertension treated. Captopril holds promise of being particularly effective for this purpose. Renal, cardiac, pulmonary, and gastrointestinal problems are managed in their own right.

Course and prognosis

The course is highly variable. Some patients progress inexorably to death from renal, pulmonary, or cardiac causes. In others the clinical course is dominated by vascular problems, especially in the fingers. Some patients run only a very slowly progressive course over many years. Occasional cases appear to remit spontaneously. Mean survival following diagnosis is about five years.

POLYARTERITIS NODOSA

Inflammatory diseases of blood vessels (vasculitis) are rare. The best known is polyarteritis nodosa (PAN). However, there is a complex classification of various named types, ranging from relatively benign skin conditions (cutaneous vasculitis) to serious systemic diseases (e.g. Goodpasture's and Wegener's syndromes). Vasculitis may also be a feature of the various systemic connective tissue diseases (Table 6.1). Thus, the most severe ('malignant') cases of rheumatoid arthritis may develop some of the features of PAN. A brief account of PAN is given here. (Giant cell arteritis is discussed in Chapter 7.)

Aetiology and pathogenesis

Much evidence suggests that the central lesion is vasculitis resulting from the deposition of circulating immune complexes in vessel walls. Once fixed there, complement becomes attached, initiating the inflammatory process. Two precipitating factors are known. One is hepatitis B virus infection and the other is hypersensitivity, particularly to drugs. The latter probably represents a benign subgroup of PAN in which the main feature is cutaneous vasculitis.

The vasculitis is segmental and patchy. The clinical features depend on the size and the distribution of the vessels involved. Full thickness destruction of a vessel wall may terminate in one of three ways:

1. *Rupture and haemorrhage.* Depending on the size of the vessel the result may vary from skin purpura to a massive cerebral haemorrhage.
2. *Occlusion of the lumen.* Distal ischaemia may range from nail fold microinfarcts to gangrene of a limb.
3. *Aneurysm formation.* These may be palpable under the skin as nodules or detected by visceral angiography.

Clinical features

Young or middle-aged males are most often affected (M : F = 3:1). There is usually a systemic disturbance with fever and malaise. Almost any structure may be affected. Skin lesions are common and include livedo reticularis (a red or purple network pattern), purpura and infarcts. Hypertension is common and there may be coronary artery ischaemia or other cardiac changes. Abdominal pain is highly characteristic and there may be ischaemia of any viscera. Renal involvement is a common cause of death. Hypertension, proteinuria and haematuria are the first signs, which may progress to renal failure. Pulmonary features include infiltrates, cavitation and asthma. The latter is often accompanied by eosinophilia (and this may represent a somewhat more benign subgroup of PAN). Cerebral vasculitis may produce a variety of neurological defects. Most common is hemiplegia or a cranial nerve palsy. Involvement of vasa nervorum leads to a highly characteristic form of peripheral neuropathy, 'mononeuritis multiplex', which has an asymmetrical and stepwise evolution. Arthralgia is common. The first attack is often serious and life-threatening. Patients who survive it may go into remission after a period of weeks or months. Subsequently there may be recurrent flares.

Investigations and diagnosis

The typical laboratory findings include a high ESR and a neutrophil leucocytosis. Patients with pulmonary involvement often have an eosinophilia (see above). Tests for rheumatoid factor and anti-nuclear antibody may be positive.

Proof of the diagnosis requires positive histology. This is best sought by biopsy of an involved structure: skin, kidney, liver or sural nerve. Coeliac angiography may be useful by revealing visceral aneurysms.

PAN may mimic a wide variety of other clinical conditions. The clue that it may underly what otherwise appears to be a typical cerebro-vascular accident or myocardial infarction may be: fever, abdominal pain, hypertension, high ESR, neutrophil leucocytosis, microscopic haematuria, eosinophilia, or mononeuritis multiplex.

Management

The presence of Australia antigen or drug hypersensitivity must be excluded as precipitating causes.

Corticosteroids, usually combined with an immunosuppressive agent such as azathioprine or cyclophosphamide, are partially effective in controlling the inflammatory component of PAN. These drugs are used in full doses during active flares. A maintenance dose of azathioprine may help to reduce the recurrent flares which sometimes follow the initial attack.

Prognosis

Cutaneous vasculitis can be a relatively benign condition, but PAN with visceral involvement carries a serious prognosis. The initial attack may progress inexorably to death, particularly from renal failure. Other cases enter a chronic phase with limited activity but they remain liable to recurrent flares.

POLYMYOSITIS AND DERMATOMYOSITIS

Inflammatory disease of skeletal muscle (polymyositis) may occur either as a rare primary disease or as part of one of the other systemic connective tissue diseases (Table 6.1). When 'pure' polymyositis is accompanied by certain skin changes it is referred to as dermatomyositis. Dermatomyositis in childhood is very rare and has some special features.

The aetiology is unknown, and a weak association with malignant disease remains unexplained. Histologically involved muscles show fibre degeneration and inflammatory cell infiltration. The evidence points to mainly cell-mediated autoimmune damage.

Clinical features

Adult females are most commonly affected (F:M = 3:1). The general pattern is of a self-limiting inflammatory illness which may last for weeks, months or years. Both the severity and the tempo are highly variable. The complaints are coloured by the fact that the muscle involvement is proximal in distribution (in contrast, for example, to the distal muscle weakness of peripheral neuropathy).

The patient usually complains of the very gradual onset of trunk and proximal limb muscle weakness. Difficulty is experienced in climbing stairs, rising from a chair, or brushing the hair. In the more acute cases there may be an initial phase of swelling and tenderness of involved muscles. Later there is wasting. Girdle muscle weakness produces a waddling gait and a positive Trendelenberg sign (sagging of the opposite side of the pelvis when standing on one leg). A useful clinical test is to get the patient to lie flat on her back with arms folded across her chest, then try to rise to a sitting position while the examiner prevents the knees lifting off the couch. Significant proximal muscle weakness makes this manoeuvre impossible. Shoulder girdle power is tested by getting the patient (standing or sitting) to hold the flexed elbows out at shoulder level and to keep them there while the examiner attempts to push them downwards.

In the important differentiation of myopathic weakness (e.g. polymyositis) from neuropathic weakness (e.g. peripheral neuropathy) the key points are:

1. Myopathic weakness is proximal, neuropathic distal.
2. In myopathy the tendon reflexes are relatively better retained (they are lost early in neuropathy because of interference with the afferent pathway).
3. Neuropathy leads to sensory loss.

In dermatomyositis the skin lesions are erythematous and scaling, and appear over the face, neck, upper arms, knuckles, and over extensor surfaces generally. The eyelids may take on a violaceous 'heliotrope' hue, while scaling over the knuckles produces characteristic 'collodion patch' lesions. The muscle changes are the same as in 'pure' polymyositis.

Oesophageal hypomotility, similar to that which occurs in systemic sclerosis (p. 84) is common. It may cause dyspepsia or may be discovered only on barium swallow in the head-down position.

Careful investigation will usually reveal some features of 'overlap' with SLE or systemic sclerosis. These may take the form of minor pulmonary or renal function changes or arthralgia. Cardiac muscle involvement may produce ECG changes. In patients over the age of 40 years there is a weak association with carcinoma.

Severe polymyositis may threaten life by spreading to involve bulbar and respiratory muscles. However, provided that the patient survives the acute phase, the inflammatory component eventually—after weeks or even months—goes into remission. This may leave the patient with varying degrees of muscle fibrosis and shortening, and sometimes telltale subcutaneous calcification. A minority of patients experience late relapses.

Dermatomyositis in childhood is very rare. It differs from the adult form in that vasculitis of muscles and viscera is prominent. Also there is a greater tendency for late deforming muscle contractures (hence the importance of specialized physiotherapy). With recovery there is often gross subcutaneous calcification.

Investigations and diagnosis

Suspicion of polymyositis comes from the characteristic history of girdle-muscle weakness without sensory symptoms. Physical signs (see above) should provide strong confirmation in all but the mildest cases. However, final proof of the diagnosis rests on three tests, two of which should be positive.

1. Raised serum creatine phosphokinase (CPK) concentrations (leakage of the enzyme from damaged muscle)
2. Electromyographic changes (characteristic findings clearly differentiate polymyositis both from neuropathy and from muscular dystrophy)
3. Histological appearance on muscle biopsy (cellular infiltration and fibre degeneration)

The ESR reflects the inflammatory component of the disease, while tests of renal or respiratory function may indicate overlap with SLE or systemic sclerosis. The serum usually contains a variety of auto-antibodies. Those directed against the antigen 'Jo1' are relatively specific for polymyositis.

Management

The first line of treatment is corticosteroids in doses sufficiently large to maintain at least respiratory and bulbar function, and to tide the patient over the active phase of the illness. This will often require high dosages (e.g. prednisolone 100 mg daily) and may have to be supplemented with an immunosuppressive drug such as azathioprine (2.5 mg/kg/day) or methotrexate (0.75 mg/kg weekly by intravenous injection). This treatment is 'titrated' against the ESR and creatine phosphokinase concentration and (particularly) the clinical state of the muscles. Once improvement starts the drugs are reduced and finally withdrawn. Respiratory and bulbar muscle weakness require the usual intensive care in their own right. As it is difficult to predict which patients may progress to severe weakness, all such cases must be managed in a hospital which has facilities for intensive care. Physiotherapy has an important role to play in preventing deformities during the acute phase and in restoring function during recovery.

Prognosis

About 15 per cent of patients die of the disease. A proportion of the remainder are left with deformities due to shortened and fibrotic muscles. Associated malginancy carries a bad prognosis.

MIXED CONNECTIVE TISSUE DISEASE

On page 76 attention was drawn to the overlap and lack of clear distinction between the various systemic connective tissue diseases as classified at present (Table 6.1). For this reason clinicians continue to seek better 'clustering' of clinical features and autoantibody markers into more useful disease categories. The 'CREST' syndrome discussed above is one such attempt. More recently 'mixed connective tissue disease' (MCTD) has been proposed as a separate disorder with its own auto-antibody marker. This claim is at present being field tested.

MCTD is defined as having clinical features which are a mixture of those of SLE, polymyositis and systemic sclerosis. The condition is relatively benign, the response to corticosteroids good, and the sero-logical marker is an antibody directed against nuclear ribonucleoprotein.

Clinical features

Most patients are young adult females, and the onset may resemble scleroderma (Raynaud's phenomenon), polymyositis (muscle weakness) or SLE (rash, arthritis or serositis). Sooner or later the clinical picture becomes a varying mixture of these three diseases. However, serious renal, psychiatric, and other visceral involvement are uncommon.

Investigations

The claim for the separate identity of MCTD rests with the presence in the serum of an autoantibody directed against nuclear ribonucleoprotein. The first clue to this is likely to be a positive test for anti-nuclear antibody in a 'speckled' pattern, and in high titre. Further testing shows the antibody to be reactive with 'extractable nuclear antigen' (ENA) which includes the specific antigen: nuclear ribonucleoprotein.

Treatment and prognosis

Once the diagnosis has been made, and provided the disease activity justifies it, corticosteroids should be started in moderate dosage (e.g. prednisolone 30 mg daily) then titrated down once a response has been obtained.

The prognosis is thought to be generally better than would be expected from a condition which is a mixture of SLE, systemic sclerosis, and polymyositis. However, neither the 'separateness' of MCTD as a disease entity, nor the long-term prognosis are established yet.

SJØGREN'S SYNDROME

Sjøgren's syndrome is defined as a clinical triad of defective tear secretion (xerophthalmia), defective salivary secretion (xerostomia) and a systemic connective tissue disease (Table 6.1, p. 76). When the dry eyes and dry mouth occur without an associated connective tissue disorder the condition is referred to as the 'sicca syndrome', or 'primary' form.

Sjøgren's syndrome is most often encountered as a troublesome extra-articular feature of rheumatoid arthritis. It may also complicate any of the other systemic connective tissue disorders, as well as autoimmune thyroid or liver disease. It is not clear whether in these circumstances the Sjøgrens features are a 'complication' of the connective tissue disease, or whether it is a separate disorder triggered by the same aetiological factors.

Primary Sjøgren's syndrome (sicca syndrome) may be a somewhat different disorder. It is associated with a wide variety of autoantibodies, a tendency to lymphproliferative changes, and a number of extraglandular features. Tissue typing also points to the primary and secondary forms being distinct.

Pathology

Affected lacrimal and salivary glands become infiltrated with plasma cells and lymphocytes, including lymphoid folicles with germinal centres. The glandular elements become atrophic, and fibrosis distorts the ducts. Duct cells proliferate to produce epi-myoepithelial islands. In the primary form there is generalized lymphoid hyperplasia, and occasionally it appears that what starts as polyclonal lymphoid hyperplasia may sometimes evolve into a (neoplastic) monoclonal B-cell proliferation. Although the brunt of the disease falls mainly on the lacrimal and salivary glands, mucus secreting glands throughout the body are affected to some extent.

Clinical features

Women are affected more often than men (F : M = 9:1). Involved glands usually remain normal in size and are not tender. However, enlargement may occur in the rare primary form. Curiously, rather than actual dryness, the patient usually notices gritty irritation and stickiness of the eyes. The dryness produces conjunctivitis, filamentary keratitis, and superficial corneal erosions. Instillation of rose Bengal or fluorescein drops and slit-lamp examination allows a confident ophthalmological diagnosis to be made.

Dryness of the mouth can be distressing by interfering with swallowing. Dry foods such as cream crackers become unmanageable, and the tongue and buccal mucosa become atrophic and sensitive. Dental disease is accelerated. Respiratory tract dryness predisposes to recurrent infections, while vaginal dryness may cause atrophic vaginitis and dyspareunia.

There may be renal complications or neoplastic changes, particularly in the primary form. Renal changes affect the tubular functions of concentration and acidification. Occasionally this progresses to the full picture of either nephrogenic diabetes insipidus or renal tubular acidosis. The rare neoplastic change consists of lymphoid hyperplasia which may progress to a malignant lymphoma (see above).

Investigations

The most striking finding is the very wide range of circulating auto-antibodies, including rheumatoid factors, (see Appendix 1). Hyper-globulinaemia is characteristic and may be extreme. Occasionally there is leucopenia or thrombocytopenia.

If histological confirmation is required this is easily obtained by buccal mucosa biopsy (a minor procedure under local anaesthetic). The mucus glands in this site accurately reflect the changes in the larger glands.

Tear secrection can be measured by Schirmer's test. A strip of 5 mm wide filter paper is hooked behind the lower eyelid and left there with the eyes lightly closed for five minutes. By that time normal tear secretion should have wetted 15 mm of the filter paper. Ophthalmological tests have been mentioned above.

Management

Treatment is symptomatic. Nothing is known to halt the progress of the disorder, and there are no effective means of increasing these exocrine secretions.

Symptomatic treatment consists of the frequent use of 1 per cent methylcellulose eye drops ('artificial tears') and glycerin mouth-washes as required. Dry eyes are particularly vulnerable to heat, dryness and wind. In these conditions considerable relief can be obtained by wearing glasses with side shields—or even goggles.

REFERENCES

Ansell, B. M. (ed) (1984). Inflammatory disorders of muscle. *Clinics in rheumatic diseases.* **10** (1). Saunders, Philadelphia.

Hughes, G. R. V. (ed) (1982). Systemic lupus erythematosus. *Clinics in rheumatic diseases.* **8** (1). Saunders, Philadelphia.

Hughes, G. R. V. (1984). Autoantibodies in lupus and its variants: experience in 100 patients. *Br. med. J.* **289**, 339–42.

Jayson, M. I. V. (1984). Systemic sclerosis: a collagen or microvascular disease? *Br. med. J.* **288**, 1855–7.

Leading article (1984). Primary and secondary Sjøgren's syndrome. *Lancet.* **ii**, 730–1.

Moutsopoulos, H. M. (1980). Sjøgren's syndrome (Sicca syndrome). *Ann. intern. Med.* **92**, 212–26.

Travers, R. L. (1979). Polyarteritis nodosa and related disorders. *Br. J. Hosp. Med.* **22**, 38–45.

7 Polymyalgia rheumatica and giant cell (temporal) arteritis

Polymyalgia rheumatica is a common and important inflammatory disorder occurring in the middle aged and elderly. The prominent features are proximal muscle aches, distressing and prolonged early morning stiffness, absence of clear evidence of arthritis, and a dramatic response to small doses of corticosteroid. *Giant cell arteritis* is a form of vasculitis which, while it may involve proximal vessels, more often presents with signs of arteritis in the territory of the carotid arteries, and may cause blindness. The vasculitis can be controlled by larger doses of corticosteroid. The reason for discussing these two conditions together is that they may occur together. The nature of this association is not understood. Whether all causes of polymyalgia rheumatica have some underlying vasculitis which is usually undetected, or whether polymyalgia rheumatica is a clinical syndrome ('reaction pattern') which may be provoked in the elderly by a number of different causes (including giant cell arteritis) is unknown. The important practical consideration is that all patients with polymyalgia rheumatica have to be managed on the assumption that they may have underlying giant cell arteritis.

POLYMYALGIA RHEUMATICA

Clinical features

Polymyalgia rheumatica is rare below the age of 50 years and it appears to have a predilection for Caucasians. Females are more commonly affected (3:1). The onset may be gradual, in which case the patient notices increasing aching of proximal muscles. Muscle pain on raising the arms above the head or climbing stairs is reminiscent of polymyositis, but there is no true muscle weakness; movements are limited only by discomfort. Most impressive is the distressing early morning stiffness. This may be so severe that the patient has to be rolled out of bed by a spouse, and then stands for a period doubled up before being able to shuffle off painfully. The morning stiffness is measured in hours.

When the patient is seen by the doctor the first impression may be that the complaints are out of proportion to the physical signs. Movements of the shoulders and hips are executed slowly and painfully, and there may be some muscle tenderness in these areas. However, obvious signs of synovitis are usually lacking, and the joints can be put through a full range of movements.

A systemic disturbance accompanies the muscle symptoms. The patient feels generally unwell, with fatigue, loss of appetite, and, particularly, mental depression. Mild fever may occur. In addition, any of the features described below under giant cell arteritis may be present.

Some cases are dramatically sudden in onset. The patient goes to bed one evening perfectly well, then awakes next morning feeling as if a calamity has struck.

The 'natural' history of polymyalgia is not known for certain. Traditional teaching is that it is a self-limiting disease which goes into remission after a year or two. However, patients in whom the disease is suppressed by corticosteroids are often unable to come off this treatment, without relapsing, for very much longer periods than this.

A highly characteristic feature is the response to corticosteroids. Administration of as little as 10 mg of prednisolone daily usually produces immediate and dramatic relief of symptoms, sometimes as promptly as overnight. This is an important diagnostic pointer.

Pathology

Despite the clear clinical and laboratory evidence of an active inflammatory process, there is little to find histologically (unless there is associated giant cell arteritis), and the mechanism of the dramatic complaints is unclear. Various imaging techniques have been employed to show that there may be evidence of proximal synovitis, affecting joints such as the sternoclavicular and acromioclavicular, but this is seldom appreciated clinically.

Investigations

Most laboratory screening tests give normal results; thus tests for rheumatoid factor, anti-nuclear and other autoantibodies are negative; enzyme and electrical test for polymyositis are normal, and X-rays do not show erosions. The blood count may show a mild anaemia, but the one outstanding abnormality is a high ESR, sometimes over 100 mm/ hour. It used to be thought that occasional cases of polymyalgia had normal ESRs. However, it is now clear that the result of this test may vary from day-to-day in these patients, and a normal result in an otherwise typical case is an indication to repeat the test. Determining the ESR is so easy that there is a case to be made for using it to screen populations of elderly patients, for example in old peoples homes, for this distressing but readily treatable condition (particularly as the complaints are so readily attributable to other causes in this age group).

Even in the absence of any clinical evidence of giant cell arteritis, 'blind' biopsy of a temporal artery will show a proportion of patients to have this form of vasculitis as well. However, as the vascular lesions are segmental, a negative biopsy does not exclude vasculitis.

Diagnosis

The florid case is unmistakable, and confirmation is obtained by a therapeutic trial of prednisolone 10–15 mg daily. Difficulty may arise in differentiating rheumatoid arthritis from polymyalgia rheumatica. Sometimes rheumatoid arthritis has a somewhat 'polymyalgic' onset. An effusion in one joint does not exclude a diagnosis of polymyalgia rheumatica, but small joint polyarthritis points to an inflammatory arthropathy. The onset of polymyositis may also mimic polymalgia rheumatica, but here the diagnostic tests of serum enzymes, electro-myography, and muscle biopsy are reliable (Chapter 6). Occasionally malignant disease (e.g. myelomatosis) may have a 'polymyalgic' onset. However, these cases do not respond as well to corticosteroid treatment, and failure to respond is an indication to seek for underlying malignancy. Table 7.1 outlines a diagnostic flow chart for patients suffering from aches and pains.

Management

From what has been said above it will be clear that management of this condition poses a therapeutic dilemma. On the one hand it is often possible to control symptoms with non-steroidal anti-inflammatory drugs, but this leaves the patient at risk of developing blindness. On the other hand, administration of corticosteroids in doses which reliably prevent vascular complications places these elderly patients on a 'collision course' for developing steroid complications, particularly osteoporotic vertebral collapse.

Against this background most clinicians treat polymyalgia rheumatica (when there is no clinical evidence of vasculitis) with small doses of corticosteroid. Starting with a therapeutic trial of prednisolone 10 to 15 mg daily, this is then tapered down to the minimum which will control symptoms and keep the ESR at or near normal. The objective is finally to withdraw the drug once the condition has 'run its course'. Patients are warned to report immediately if they develop any of the symptoms of vasculitis (see below).

If this should happen, the dose is immediately increased to that appropriate for giant cell arteritis.

Opinions differ about the indications for 'blind' temporal-artery

Table 7.1. *Diagnostic flow chart: some causes of diffuse aches and pains*

Diffuse aches and pains				
	Elevated ESR	Joint pains	Marked early morning stiffness	→ Inflammatory polyarthritis (Rheumatoid, ankylosing spondylitis, psoriatic etc.)
			ANA positive	→ SLE
		Muscle and bone pain	Marked early morning stiffness	→ Polymyagia rheumatica
			Bone tenderness	→ Myelomatosis Secondary carcinoma
			Muscle weakness	→ Polymositis
	Normal ESR	Elevated alkaline phosphatase	Metabolic bone disease (Osteomalacia, Paget's, hyperparathyroidism, renal osteodystrophy)	
			Secondary carcinoma (*)	
		Normal alkaline phosphatase	Generalized osteoarthritis	
			Spondylosis	
			Osteoporosis	
			Secondary carcinoma (*)	
			Fibrositis (**)	
			Psychogenic	

(*)Secondary carcinomatous deposits may or may not cause elevation of the serum alkaline phosphatase.

(**)'Fibrositis' is a term used by some clinicians to describe a syndrome of diffuse muscular aches associated with tender 'trigger points' for which no cause can be found. It is not an established disease entity.

biopsy. The yield is generally low in patients without clinical evidence of vasculitis and a negative biopsy does not exclude it. However, some feel that the late difficulties of maintaining elderly patients on long-term steroids are so great that every advantage should be taken to make the diagnosis as secure as possible (before corticosteroids obscure the evidence). Under local anaesthetic the procedure is very minor.

Some of the problems in management are best illustrated by a case history:

Mrs G, aged 65, had seldom troubled her doctor. Apart from a previous episode of 'frozen shoulder' following herpes zoster, and occasional neck and arm pains, diagnosed as cervical spondylosis and helped by wearing a collar, she remained active and sprightly. Then, two weeks previously, her 'life had changed'. She experienced increasing aches in her neck, shoulders and buttocks, and awoke each morning with crippling morning stiffness which lasted until mid-morning. She felt generally unwell, depressed, and had lost her appetite.

Physical examination revealed tenderness of shoulder girdle muscles and buttocks, but no definite arthritis. Joint movements were executed reluctantly, but the range was full. Her breasts were normal, and general physical examination otherwise negative.

Investigations yielded a negative latex and anti-nuclear antibody test, and a normal alkaline phosphatase concentration. The blood count was unremarkable, but the ESR was elevated at 80 mm/hour.

As the evidence pointed to a diagnosis of polymyalgia rheumatica, an attempt was made to get her into hospital overnight for a temporal artery biopsy, but no bed was available. After a telephone consultation with a rheumatologist, her doctor reviewed the question of whether there was any evidence of underlying giant cell arteritis. In the absence of headache, visual disturbance, scalp and tenderness, facial pain, or jaw claudication it was concluded that there was none, so she was immediately started on prednisolone 15 mg daily.

Next day she was dramatically improved and within 48 hours was completely free of pain and back to her usual cheerful self. The ESR fell to 18 mm/hour within a week, and a chest X-ray was normal.

Over the following months the dose of prednisolone was gradually titrated down. She required about 8 mg daily (using 1 mg tablets for fine adjustment) in order to prevent muscle pains and keep her sedimentation rate below 20 mm/hour. On two occasions the dose was temporarily increased to 30 mg daily, once because of the appearance of headaches, and once because of rather vague facial pain.

Two years after the onset it was proving very difficult to reduce the dose of prednisolone below 7.5 mg daily without provoking vague skeletal pains. Mrs G was by now somewhat Cushingoid, mildly hypertensive and had developed dyspepsia. Her ESR was 25 mm/hour. Her doctor and the rheumatologist were beginning to feel that her interests might now best be served by reducing the dose of prednisolone further, despite some myalgic symptoms, but continuing to monitor for any more definite evidence of arteritis. It was agreed that if prednisolone could not be stopped, and dyspepsia continued, it would be necessary to arrange for gastroscopy or a barium meal, and consider the introduction of cimetidine.

GIANT CELL ARTERITIS (TEMPORAL OR CRANIAL ARTERITIS)

Clinical features

Women are affected more than men, and most patients are over the age of 50 years. Systemic complaints are common, with malaise, mild fever and—in some patients—polymyalgia rheumatica (see above).

The most common symptom of vasculitis is headache. This may be severe and persistent, and either generalized or limited to one area of the scalp. There may be local scalp tenderness and, particularly over the temporal arteries, a local segment of inflamed artery may be felt as a tender cord with a visible redness and overlying oedema. Pressure of the pillow at night may make it feel like 'lying on a marble'. On examination the prominent vessel lacks pulsation. Occipital or other scalp vessels may become involved.

Similar pains may become experienced in the side of the face, the jaw, or on one side of the tongue. Gangrene of part of the tongue has been described. A highly characteristic complaint is claudication in the muscles of mastication during eating.

The most serious manifestation of this disease is ophthalmic arteritis. Diplopia, blurring of vision or eye pain may give some warning, but blindness can be sudden, bilateral and complete, owing to occlusion of the retinal artery.

Arteritis of other intracranial vessels may produce a variety of clinical pictures, including hemiplegia, epilepsy and psychosis.

Post-mortem studies show that large vessels such as the aorta are also involved. Occasionally these patients may present with an 'aortic-arch' syndrome, including loss of peripheral pulses. This appears to be a separate condition from the pathologically similar Takayasu's artertitis which occurs in younger women.

Investigations

The characteristic laboratory finding is a markedly elevated ESR, often over 100 mm/hour. Biopsy of a clinically involved temporal artery shows a necrotizing vasculitis with fragmentation of the internal elastic lamina, and collections of giant cells.

Management

As soon as the diagnosis is made, and if the clinical features point only to the involvement of the scalp vessels, corticosteroid treatment is started as prednisolone 60 mg daily. However, if there are features suggesting intra-cranial involvement then the minimum starting dose is 100 mg daily. Biopsy confirmation is sought as soon as possible, but steroid therapy is not delayed for this (a day or two of steroid treatment does not destroy the histological evidence).

Full doses of prednisolone are maintained for about three weeks, then the dose is gradually reduced to the minimum that will keep the patient free of symptoms and the ESR normal. Reappearance of arteritis symptoms is an indication for an immediate increase in dosage. Eventually it should be possible to withdraw corticosteroids, but this can take several years. Late recurrences may occur.

REFERENCES

Dixon, A. St J. (1983). Polymyalgia rheumatica. In *Reports on rheumatic diseases: Collected reports: 1958–1983.* Arthritis and Rheumatism Council, London.

Hazleman, B. (1976). Giant cell arteritis and polymyalgia rheumatica. In *Modern Topics in Rheumatology.* Hughes, G. R. V. (ed). Heinemann, London.

Jones, J. G. and Hazleman, B. L. (1981). Prognosis and management of poly-myalgia rheumatica. *Ann. Rheum. Dis.* **40**, 1–5.

8 Infective arthritis

Infections may cause, or be related to, arthritis in a number of different ways. At one end of the scale is the situation in which an organism such as a *Staphylococcus* species or tubercle bacillus invades the joint tissues to cause inflammation and damage. At the other end there is unproven speculation that micro-organisms, perhaps viruses, play some role in the pathogenesis of diseases such as rheumatoid arthritis, SLE, and Behçet's syndrome. Between these two extremes is a group of disorders in which a definite infection is followed by arthritis due, not to direct invasion of the joint tissues by the infecting agent, but to the interplay of organisms and host immunological response. Examples of this include rheumatic fever, Reiter's disease and other conditions referred to as 'reactive arthritis' (p. 60), as well as some arthropathies which follow virus infections. Some infections may operate in both ways, such that both direct local invasion and immunolgical reactions contribute to the arthritis. Examples of this are thought to be neisserial infections with meningococci or gonococci. This chapter is devoted mainly to the types of infective arthritis caused by direct invasion of the joint. These conditions are not common, but their recognition is critical. Mis-diagnosis or mis-managment can result in joint destruction and a threat to life.

SUPPURATIVE (PYOGENIC) ARTHRITIS

Primary invasion of the joint is rare in the absence of some predisposing cause. General predisposing causes include anything which lowers resistance to infection (immunosuppression, malignant disease, etc.), pyaemia from any cause (intravenous catheters, bacterial endocarditis, intravenous drug abuse, etc.), while local factors include implanted artificial joints, penetrating injuries, or the presence of other types of joint damage, particularly rheumatoid arthritis. Bed sores or urinary tract infections may provide the source of entry of infection via the bloodstream. The extreme rarity of infection complicating therapeutic joint aspiration and/or corticosteroid injection is testimony to the high level of natural resistance to bacterial infection, even in diseased joints.

Pathology

The commonest micro-organisms involved in adult joint infections are the staphylococci, streptococci and gonococci. Children may be infected by *Haemophilus influenzae* or Gram-negative bacilli as well. In patients with sickle cell anaemia infections with *Salmonella* species are particularly common. Immunosuppressed patients may become infected with organisms which are not normally pathogenic, while intravenous drug abuse may result in joint invasion by unusual organisms.

The invaded synovium becomes intensely hyperaemic and densely invaded with neutrophil leucocytes. The synovial effusion is at first serous, then purulent. From this stage onwards enzymatic digestion progressively softens and destroys the articular cartilage, while granulation tissue grows out from the synovial margin into the joint. With healing this may produce fibrous ankylosis. Subchondral bone becomes porotic and there may be osteolysis and, with healing, osteosclerosis, or even bony ankylosis. Early antimicrobial treatment can cut short this process and allow the joint to return to normal. A neglected joint may be the source of pyaemic spread of infection to other sites.

Clinical findings

Any age group may be infected. The classical presentation of (rare) 'primary' pyogenic joint infection is the development, over twenty-four hours, of a very acutely inflamed, painful, stiff and swollen joint. The pain is constant and distressing, and there are likely to be systemic features of fever and malaise. However, in elderly and debilitated patients, and particularly in those taking corticosteroid drugs, these features may be much less dramatic. Any joint in the body may become infected, but the most common sites are the large or medium-sized articulations, particularly the knee.

On examination the skin over a septic joint is often red (erythema is uncommon over uncomplicated rheumatoid joints; it is generally evidence of more acute inflammation such as crystal synovitis, Reiter's disease, or sepsis). The infected joint is likely to be distended by an effusion and (in order to minimize the pain of synovial distension) is held in the position which provides maximum volume within the synovial cavity. In the knee and hip joints this is a position of partial flexion. There is usually extreme tenderness over the joint surface, while both active and passive movements may be too painful to perform. As stated previously, in the elderly, the debilitated, and patients taking corticosteroid drugs these signs and symptoms may be less dramatic.

An important aspect of this physical examination is to differentiate between inflammation close to, but outside, the joint cavity and septic arthritis within the joint itself. Acute pre- or infrapatellar bursitis may, on superficial examination, be mistaken for septic arthritis of the knee joint. Careful palpation, however, will show that the extreme tenderness is all anterior, while the joint line on either side is unaffected. Similarly, while full flexion of the knee joint will—by distorting soft tissues—produce pain, a relatively painless middle range of movement should be obtainable. Such peri-articular inflammation may produce a 'sympathetic' effusion in the nearby joint. In these circumstances it is particularly important to avoid passing a needle through the infected soft tissues into the sterile joint.

Investigations

An elevated ESR and a neutrophil leucocytosis reflect the presence of a pyogenic infection. The responsible organism can often be grown from the peripheral blood, and both blood and synovial fluid should be obtained for culture before any antibiotics are given. Examination of the synovial fluid is important and must never be postponed or delayed if septic arthritis is suspected.

Traditionally septic arthritis yields a 'purulent' synovial fluid. In fact, this is so only when the condition is well established. In the early stages the fluid may be serous. Further, non-infected rheumatoid joints may sometimes yield fluids which appear purulent. Purulent fluids contain $50-300 \times 10^9/1$ leucocytes and over 90 per cent of these are neutrophils. A Gram stain may give a valuable lead about the presence of bacteria, but both culture and sensitivity tests are essential. X-rays are normal in the early stages. Later the peri-articular bone becomes porotic and cartilage destruction is revealed as a loss of joint space. In spinal infections there may be loss of disc space (Fig. 8.1).

Diagnosis

A variety of arthropathies and peri-articular conditions can present a picture sufficiently acute to raise the possibility of infection. These include:

Acute gout or pyrophosphate arthropathy.
Reiter's disease.
Cellulitis.
Acute prepatellar bursitis.
Palindromic rheumatism.
Acute rheumatic fever.
Sickle cell crisis.
Haemophilic joint bleed.

Particular care is necessary to avoid missing the development of septic arthritis in a patient with rheumatoid arthritis. This is especially so in those taking corticosteroid drugs since the signs and symptoms of infection may be suppressed. Thus, when a single joint becomes more painful and inflamed it is usually advisable to aspirate it. An even more difficult problem is that of identifying infection in a joint containing a prosthesis. Suspicion of this (pain, fever or a discharging wound) is an indication for a referral to an orthopaedic unit. Radiology and isotopic scanning can provide pointers to the presence of low-grade infection, but at present this remains an area of considerable diagnostic difficulty.

Management

Septic arthritis is a serious condition which requires immediate transfer of the patient to hospital. The first requirement is to aspirate the joint and take blood cultures. Specimens from immunosuppressed patients and intravenous drug abusers require special processing and the laboratory should be warned in advance.

> Patients in whom septic arthritis is suspected must never be given antimicrobial drugs before blood and joint fluid have been obtained for laboratory examination.

The patient is put to bed and the affected joint rested by splinting. In the knee this is best achieved by a Thomas' splint with light traction. Strong analgesics may be needed. It is important to remove joint fluid as it accumulates. This is done by daily aspiration (occasionally more often). If loculation occurs it is usual to undertake arthrotomy, break down loculating adhesions, and establish closed drainage by suction.

Early, appropriate, and aggressive antimicrobial therapy is needed. Antibiotics enter the inflamed joint space readily, so there is normally no need to inject them locally into the joint (indeed they may be irritant).

Antibiotic therapy cannot wait for complete microbiological investigation. Broad-spectrum treatment is started while waiting for precise identification of the bacterium and its sensitivity pattern. The result of the initial Gram stain may provide a useful pointer to the likely organism. The following guidelines may be followed:

1. Presumed staphylococcal: Flucloxacillin, nafcillin, clindamycin or fucidin (in children under 3 years of age add ampicillin in case of *H. influenzae* infection).
2. Presumed *Psuedomonas* species or other Gram-negative rods: Gentamicin combined with carbenicillin or ticarcillin.
3. Presumed gonococcal: Penicillin G.

More precise indentification of the bacterium and the pattern of its sensitivity allow the antimicrobial therapy to be tailored. Generally the drugs are given in full doses parenterally for the first week, then orally for a further three weeks or longer. The total duration of therapy will depend on the rate of clinical improvement, the rate at which the effusion clears, and the characteristics of the fluid at sequential aspirations (including repeated bacteriological cultures). The strategy of antimicrobial therapy is best planned in conjunction with the microbiologist.

Muscle-strengthening exercises are started as soon as the acute inflammation settles, and these are followed by active and passive joint movements as soon as possible. Provided treatment is started before irreversible damage has occurred (a few days in acute cases), the final outcome is usually satisfactory. Inadequate or delayed treatment is likely to result in residual stiffness and later secondary osteoarthritis. Failure to treat septic arthritis (e.g. in a rheumatoid patient taking corticosteroids) can result in fatal septicaemia.

GONOCOCCAL ARTHRITIS

Pyogenic arthritis resulting from gonococcal infection has features in common with those of septic arthritis described above, but there are some interesting and important differences. Most of these apply also to the much less common meningococcal arthritis, and thus appear to be characteristic of neisserial infections in general.

Something like 1 per cent of patients with sexually-acquired gonococcal infections develop systemic features of 'disseminated gonococcal infection' (DGI). For reasons which are not clear, this proportion appears to be much higher in North America than in Britain. Nevertheless, because gonorrhoea is so common in both countries, it accounts for a considerable proportion of cases of pyogenic arthritis amongst the sexually active. Factors which determine whether gonococcal infections become disseminated include the strain of the organism, the integrity of the complement system (complement-deficient subjects are more susceptible), and sex, women being ten times more liable to DGI. This may be due to the local infection being less obvious (and hence neglected) in females, or to other factors; for example, the onset of DGI is commoner during menstruation or pregnancy.

There is evidence that there may be more than one pathological mechanism operating in gonococcal arthritis. The observation that the arthritis is sometimes 'flitting' and may resolve without treatment, and the fact that fluid from affected joints is often sterile, point to mechanisms other than straightforward bacterial invasion. Suggested mechanisms include circulating immune complexes producing a 'serum sickness', chemical synovitis from non-viable gonococcal material, or a form of reactive arthritis (p. 60).

Clinical features

The interval between sexual exposure and the onset of DGI is highly variable (days to weeks). The first evidence of dissemination is generally malaise and fever, followed by the appearance of arthritis which may migrate from one joint to another, or settle in one site to produce the picture of septic arthritis (see above). A common and characteristic feature is the appearance of tenosynovitis, particularly in finger tendon sheaths. At some stage a skin rash develops. This may pass unnoticed by the patient, but is highly characteristic of DGI. These lesions are most common on the limbs. Starting as 1 to 2 mm violaceous papules, they evolve into vesicular, haemorrhagic or pustular lesions which do not itch. More serious features of DGI are endocarditis, meningitis or peri-hepatitis. Untreated, a migratory arthritis may resolve spontaneously or settle in one joint to give the picture of septic arthritis. Even this may settle without residual damage (as commonly happened in pre-antibiotic days), but sometimes there is joint destruction. When penicillin is administered the response is usually dramatic; complete resolution occurs within a few days.

Management

When DGI is suspected microbiological investigations should include joint fluid and blood cultures, as well as urethral, cervical, pharyngeal, and rectal cultures. The skin lesions are generally sterile.

Organisms responsible for DGI are almost invariably sensitive to penicillin. A typical regimen is to give 10 million units of penicillin G, intravenously, daily until symptoms subside, then oral ampicillin 2 g daily for a total of 10 days.

General managment includes tracing contacts and screening for other sexually-acquired diseases, and this is usually best undertaken by a specialist in genitourinary medicine.

TUBERCULOUS ARTHRITIS

Skeletal tuberculosis is always secondary to a focus elsewhere, and it generally involves the joint and adjacent bone simultaneously. The disease is becoming uncommon amongst Caucasians, but it remains an important form of arthritis in most parts of Africa, Asia and South America. In Britain most cases are seen amongst Asian immigrants.

Clinical features

Children and young adults are most often affected, although any age may be involved. Tuberculosis has a predilection for the spinal and weight-bearing joints (hip, knee and ankle).

The presentation is less acute than with the septic arthritis, and the patient usually describes weeks or months of vague ill health, often with mild fever, night sweats and loss of weight. One, two or a few joints may be involved. The inflammation is less acute than that in a septic joint (see above), but rather more acute than a rheumatoid joint. When the spine is involved (Pott's disease) an extremely important sign is local tenderness over the spinous process of the affected vertebra.

A highly characteristic feature of tuberculous infections is a tendency for them to track for long distances and present as 'cold abscesses' at a site remote from the original focus. Thus vertebral infections may track down the sheath of the psoas muscle to present in the femoral triangle of the thigh, or track around a rib under the periosteum to present as a fluctuant swelling over the anterior chest wall. Mild pyrexia is common.

Investigations

The ESR is usually raised and a mild anaemia is common. An important point is that the chest X-ray is often normal (implying that the portal of entry was via the tonsil or gut), but the Mantoux test is generally positive, often strongly so. Synovial fluid from an affected joint may yield acid-fast bacilli, but this is frequently negative. It usually requires histology from a synovial biopsy in order to make a confident diagnosis. Sometimes there is no alternative to carrying out a therapeutic trial using anti-tuberculous drugs. However, full bacteriological identification and sensitivity testing is desirable. A similar clinical and radiological picture may be produced by atypical mycobacterial infections, fungal arthritis or brucellosis. (The last is a rare cause of arthritis in British holidaymakers returning from Spain).

X-rays of an affected joint may be normal in the early stages. Sometimes a lucent area in an adjacent bone indicates a peri-articular bone focus. Over a period of weeks local rarefaction develops as does a loss of 'joint space' as the cartilage is destroyed. The radiological signs in the spine are characteristic of joint infections generally. Typically there is partial collapse of a vertebral body with loss of the adjacent intervertebral disc spaces (Fig. 8.1). This last feature distinguishes spinal infections from vertebral collapse due to neoplasms (e.g. secondary deposits from a breast carcinoma, in which case the disc spaces are preserved). Additional features are a fusiform shadow indicating an abscess and loss of the outline of the psoas muscle. Multiple spinal levels may be involved.

Management

While awaiting sensitivity tests the patient is generally given triple anti-tuberculous therapy (rifampicin, isoniazid, and ethambutol). Once the organism's sensitivity is known treatment is continued with two drugs. Treatment may be needed for three to six months.

Normal	Neoplasia	Infection

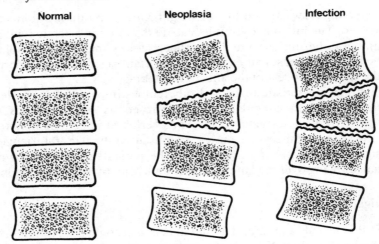

Fig. 8.1. Diagram comparing the radiological changes in the spine when collapse of a vertebra results from a secondary deposit or an infection (e.g. tuberculosis). The distinguishing feature is the loss of adjacent intervertebral disc spaces in the case of infection, and their preservation in the case of malignant deposits.

In the spine operative surgery may be called for to drain an abscess, relieve pressure on the contents of the spinal canal, or to fuse unstable segments. A bonus from doing this is that it provides material for culture and sensitivity testing and allows confirmation of the diagnosis. Similarly synovectomy of the peripheral joints may be undertaken.

The outlook is excellent provided adequate treatment is given in good time. Neglected spinal tuberculosis can lead to very gross 'gibbous' angulation (probably the common cause of the 'hunchback' deformities of previous times) and paraplegia.

VIRAL ARTHRITIS

A variety of virus infections may produce a self-limiting episode of polyarthritis. Often the features of the causative infection are so mild as to pass unnoticed and, unless serial antibody studies are undertaken, the cause of the arthritis is never discovered. The organisms involved include those responsible for rubella, type-B hepatitis, chicken pox, mumps and infectious mononucleosis. Less commonly, a wide variety of other virus infections may be followed by arthritis.

The pathogenesis of these arthropathies is not yet established for certain, and this may vary between the different organisms. Possible mechanisms include direct synovial invasion, a type of immune-complex 'serum sickness', virus-induced autoimmunity, or 'reactive arthritis' (p. 60).

The best studied form of viral arthritis is rubella. This is usually seen in young adult females. It may follow a natural infection (often atypical or mild and unnoticed) or active vaccination. Arthritis may develop before, during, or after the appearance of a rubella exanthem. The joint symptoms vary in severity from a mild polyarthritis lasting a week or two, to a more persistent arthropathy resembling rheumatoid arthritis and lasting for many months. There has been speculation that rubella may occasionally be the trigger for progressive rheumatoid arthritis, but this is not established. Tenosynovitis and carpal tunnel syndrome may complicate rubella arthritis. Histological changes in the synovium are inconspicuous, but the virus can occasionally be cultured from the joint, In the absence of a history of a rubella rash or exposure to infection, the diagnosis is established by a rising antibody titre. Treatment is symptomatic. Occasionally a short course of corticosteroids may be given to cut short the arthritis.

Arthritis may be the presenting feature of hepatitis-B infection. A mild and transient polyarthritis appears at the same time as an urticarial skin eruption. This is due to a pre-icteric phase of circulating immune complexes producing a 'serum sickness'.

SPIROCHAETAL ARTHRITIS

Clutton's joints are painful knee or elbow effusions occurring in teenage children with congenital syphilis.

Secondary syphilis may be complicated by mild polyarthritis probably caused by circulating immune complexes.

Lyme disease is a spirochaetal infection recently described in Connecticut. It is transmitted by a tick. The multi-system disorder causes polyarthritis in 60 per cent of patients. This occasionally becomes chronic and destructive.

REFERENCES

Goldenberg, D. L. and Cohen, A. S. (1976). Acute infectious arthritis. *Am. J. Med.* **60**, 369–77.

Halsey, J. P., Reeback, J. S., and Barnes, C. G. (1982). A decade of skeletal tuberculosis. *Ann. Rheum. Dis.* **41**, 7–10.

Jessop, J. D. (1983). Joint infections. In *reports on rheumatic diseases: collected reports: 1958–1983*, pp. 81–3. Arthritis and Rheumatism Council, London.

Manshady, B. M., Thompson, G. R., and Weiss, J. J. (1980). Septic arthritis in a general hospital. *J. Rheumatol.* **7**, 523–70.

Masi, A. T. and Eisenstein, B. I. (1981). Disseminated gonococcal infection (DGI) and gonococcal arthritis (GCA): II. Clinical manifestations, diagnosis, complications, treatment and prevention. *Seminars in arthritis and rheumatism* **10**, 173–97. Saunders, Philadelphia.

9 Other diseases with joint manifestations

Collected together in this chapter are various conditions in which arthritis forms part of the clinical picture. They are listed here in alphabetical order, not in order of importance. Futher examples of this will be found in the chapter on systemic connective tissue diseases (Chapter 6).

BEHÇET'S SYNDROME

This term is applied to a rare symptom complex which includes particularly painful mouth and genital ulcers, and inflammatory eye disease, usually iritis. Its cause is not established and indeed it is not known whether this constitutes a true disease entity. Other features which may occur include inflammatory polyarthritis, neurological lesions, and thrombophlebitis. No treatment is reliably effective, although corticosteroids and immunosuppressive drugs are often tried.

ERYTHEMA NODOSUM

Erythema nodosum is a clinical syndrome in which the central feature is a characteristic skin eruption. It may result from a variety of causes, including:

Infections: streptococcal throats, tuberculosis, leprosy, etc.
Drugs: sulphonamides, bromides.
Other diseases: sarcoidosis, inflammatory bowel disease, neoplasia.
Pregnancy and the contraceptive pill.

Whatever the precipitating cause (and this may never be discovered) the full 'reaction pattern' may include malaise, fever, a high ESR, and arthralgia or true arthritis.

The skin lesions characteristically appear as tender red swellings down the front of the shins, less often on other extensor surfaces. They remain for a few days then begin to fade and become less tender. As they fade they pass through the yellow/greenish colours characteristic of a bruise. Recurrent crops may appear. While the skin lesions are active the patient may experience considerable malaise and fever, and—in a proportion of cases—joint symptoms. These range from arthralgia to acute inflammatory arthritis. Usually the joints of the lower limb are affected, particularly the ankles. It can be difficult to tell whether erythema over the ankles is part of the arthritis or an overlying skin lesion. The skin lesions never break down, and both they and the arthritis (when present) resolve over a few weeks.

Management includes rest and symptomatic treatment with non-steroidal anti-inflammatory drugs. However, the main responsibility is to establish the underlying cause. In Britain the common associations are streptococcal sore throats, tuberculosis, drugs and a benign form of sarcoidosis (see below) known as Lofgren's syndrome. This occurs mainly in young women and consists of erythema nodosum, polyarthritis, and hilar lymphadenopathy (identified on chest X-ray). The prognosis for complete recovery is excellent.

The pathogenesis of the skin lesions is not understood, but is probably immunological. The likelihood of arthritis occurring, and its severity, appear to be independent of the precipitating cause—except in the case of leprosy, which tends to be associated with particularly severe skin and joint lesions ('erythema nodosum leprosum').

HAEMOPHILIA

Both true haemophilia (lack of factor VIII) and Christmas disease (lack of factor IX) are inherited as sex-linked recessive genetic defects and thus affect boys exclusively. Those with less than 2 per cent of the normal levels of either of these factors are likely to suffer from recurrent bleeds, and joints are one of the most common sites of bleeding.

An acute haemarthrosis (or occasionally a visit to the dentist) is the common manner of presentation of haemophilia in a young boy. The bleed may be spontaneous or precipitated by minor trauma. The blood distends the synovial cavity to produce an acutely painful joint (the pain is due to distension of the joint capsule, perhaps combined with some irritant action of the blood). Untreated the joint remains painful for some days, or weeks. A particularly distressing feature, however, is the propensity for recurrence of bleeding to occur when he attempts to use the joint again.

Generally, larger joints such as the knee or elbow are involved, and there may be associated peri-articular bleeding which can cause diagnostic confusion. Soft tissue bleeds are painful, but generally not as acute as intra-articular haemorrhages. Soft tissue bleeds are particularly hazardous when they occur in confined spaces such as the groin and cause pressure on the nerves and blood vessels.

Recurrent haemarthroses render joints more liable to further bleeds. In time there may develop a proliferative synovitis which somewhat resembles a chronic rheumatoid joint. A knee joint involved in this manner becomes a severe handicap since the patients suffers chronic pain and disability punctuated by episodes of acute and painful bleeds.

The pain of acute attacks is so severe that the boys are in danger of becoming addicted to powerful analgesic drugs.

Management

Optimal treatment is critical. Mismanagement of early bleeds can lead to a lifetime of pain and disability.

Every haemophiliac must be registered with a local haemophilia centre. His management is then a combined operation between the centre, the general practitioner and the family. The basis of treatment is replacement therapy. Concentrated extracts of both factors VIII and IX are now available, but all these have to be given intravenously. The treatment of an acute bleed is immediate replacement of the missing factor, rest for the joint, analgesia (avoiding intramuscular injections which may themselves cause bleeding), followed by gradual mobilization, and muscle-strengthening exercises. Meanwhile, sufficient replacement therapy should be given to prevent recurrent bleeding. Most authorities favour aspiration of the joint (under adequate replacement of the missing factor) when an effusion is tense.

Early treatment is so important in all haemophiliac crises that it is appropriate to give replacement therapy before establishing the diagnosis. Thus, whether it be a probable bleed into a joint or an 'acute abdomen' it is essential to give immediate replacement before undertaking any diagnostic steps. For this the patient must have open access to a nearby hospital able to provide replacement therapy. The specific arrangements will depend on local circumstances, and are a matter for planning between the haemophilia centre, the patient and his family, and the general practitioner. Joint bleeds of any severity require admission to hospital, not least because of the need for expert physiotherapy, splinting etc. Occasionally a chronic, badly damaged joint causes so much pain and disability that synovectomy or some other surgical procedures is undertaken. The logistics of the replacement therapy involved are daunting, but not impossible.

Really effective therapy awaits the development of a preparation (ideally one taken orally) which can be used for prophylaxis. Until that becomes possible, reliance will have to be placed on the available intravenous preparations. These introduce hazards of immunological intolerance and infection (hepatitis B, AIDS etc.), and impose great demands on health services.

HAEMOGLOBINOPATHIES

Congenital haemoglobin abnormalities such as sickle cell anaemia may produce gross bony abnormalities, including aseptic necrosis of the femoral head and other changes which produce skeletal pains. The gross abnormalities occur particularly in the severely affected homozygotes. However, heterozygotes with the 'trait' may also suffer lesser skeletal pains. For this reason, rheumatological complaints among immigrants to Britain, particularly those coming from the West Indies or Africa, are an indication for haemoglobin screening.

In patients with sickle cell disease the rheumatological complaints will usually appear against a background of more general ill health, including anaemia, splenomegaly, jaundice, leg ulcers, infections (including osteitis and septic arthritis), and sometimes renal failure. Infants may present with the 'hand-and-foot syndrome' of painful dactylitis with swelling of the fingers and feet. The most dramatic manifestions likely to be encountered are the 'crises' which manifest themselves as skeletal pains.

These episodes may be precipitated by cold, anoxia, or infection, and are thought to result from thrombotic vascular occlusions. On X-ray there may be evidence of bone infarcts, but the most characteristic rheumatological complication is aseptic necrosis of the head of the femur, or sometimes of the humerus.

The crises can be excessively painful, and all but the mildest episodes require admission to hospital. Unfortunately no specific treatment is available, and management consists of treating any infection, and giving intravenous fluids, oxygen and analgesics. Occasionally, exchange transfusions are employed.

HENOCH–SCHÖNLEIN PURPURA (ANAPHYLACTOID PURPURA)

Like erythema nodosum (see above) anaphylactoid purpura appears to be a reaction pattern, one component of which is usually polyarthritis. The condition is named after the characteristic skin lesions. Other features include abdominal pain, sometimes more serious intestinal complications, and glomerulonephritis. The condition is most common in children and usually follows an upper respiratory tract infection. The syndrome appears to result from widespread vasculitis, perhaps caused by circulating immune complexes. The presence of IgA in renal mesangial cells suggests that there may be a relationship with other forms of renal disease having this feature.

The skin lesions are highly characteristic. They occur on the buttocks and extensor surfaces of the limbs. The actual purpuric spot is situated in the centre of a raised erythematous papule, and is quite unlike the (impalpable) purpura due to thrombocytopenia. There may also be urticaria and abdominal colic, and, rarely, intestinal haemorrhage or intussesception. About half the patients develop acute glomerulo-nephritis, but only a small proportion progress to chronic renal disease.

The arthritis consists of a transient synovitis affecting, particularly, the ankles, knees, hips, wrists, and elbows. This usually settles within a month, and treatment is symptomatic. Rarely steroids may be given for treatment for intestinal problems. These patients require follow-up for a few months to make sure that they are not left with residual or progressive renal disease.

HYPERMOBILITY

There is considerable variation in the range of joint movements between different individuals. Greater mobility is normally found in the young, in females, and in members of races with pigment in their skin. In addition, certain rare genetic diseases of connective tissue (Marfan's and Ehlers–Danlos syndromes) may be associated with extreme hypermobility. These latter subjects tend to develop a variety of joint complaints, including low back ache, and are also liable to premature degenerative joint disease.

In addition to this there is evidence that those individuals at the upper range of 'normal' mobility (the type of person regarded as being 'double-jointed') are to some extent also more liable to articular problems. It is therefore useful to have a yardstick by which to judge joint mobility. The tests shown in Figure 9.1 serve this purpose. Four of the five tests are paired, and each positive test is given a score of one, making a possible total of nine. Scores of five or greater indicate 'hypermobility'.

This raises the question of the advice that should be given regarding exercise programmes. It would appear reasonable to endorse the value of exercises such as swimming and cycling, which improve muscle strength without stretching the joints, but to advise against exercises aimed at increasing the range of joint movements beyond the normal limits (e.g. 'doing the splits').

METABOLIC BONE DISEASES

Generalized diseases of the skeleton may sometimes lead to arthritis. More often they cause skeletal pains which may closely mimic rheumatic diseases, and the correct diagnosis is then easily overlooked. The brief notes which follow are included to draw attention to the need to consider these conditions in the differential diagnosis of 'rheumatic' complaints (Table 9.1).

Osteoporosis (Osteopenia)

Skeletal mass normally increases up to the age of about 35 years, after which the bones gradually become thinner. Sex hormones influence this

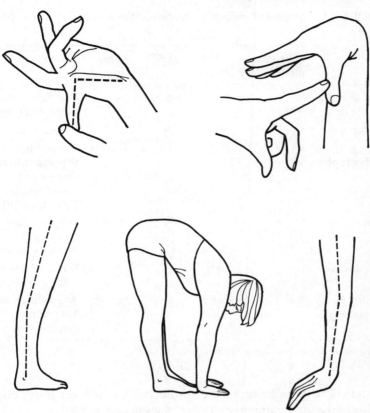

Fig. 9.1. Tests for hypermobility. Elbow and knee hyperextension are positive when 10 degrees or greater; little finger hyperextension is positive if 90 degrees or greater. Wrist flexion counts as positive if the thumb can be made to touch the forearm. As four of the tests are paired, the possible total score is nine. Subjects scoring five or more are regarded as 'hypermobile'.

process and significant osteoporosis is a disorder mainly of post-menopausal females. It is very common. Other causes include immobility (lack of mechanical stress), intestinal malabsorption, thyrotoxicosis, and, particularly, the administration of corticosteroids.

Uncomplicated osteoporosis is probably not in itself painful. Pain occurs once one of the thinned bones fractures. Such fractures are most common at the wrist (Colles' fracture), the neck of the femur, and the bodies of the lower dorsal and upper lumbar vertebrae. Corticosteroid therapy causes (mainly) medullary bone thinning and results in vertebral crush fractures. The precipitating trauma involved may be minimal. Thus, an elderly woman in stepping off a pavement may jolt herself slightly and

Table 9.1. *Some useful pointers in the differential diagnosis of bone diseases*

	Alkaline phosphatase	Serum calcium	ESR	Other tests	X-rays
Osteoporosis	N	N	N	—	Cod-fish vertebrae Crush fractures
Osteomalacia	↑	N or ↓	N	Vit D ↓	Pseudo-fractures
Renal osteodystrophy	↑	↓↑	↑	B Urea ↑	Mixture of hyperparathyroid disease and osteomalacia Ectopic calcification
Hyperpara-thyroidism	↑	↑	N	PTH ↑	Subperiosteal erosions 'Brown tumours'
Paget's disease	↑	N(*)	N	—	Widened bones Coarse trabeculae
Multiple myelomatosis	N or ↑	↑ or N	↑	Ig ↑	'Moth-eaten' bones May mimic osteoporosis

(*) Raised if patient immobilized in bed.

immediately be gripped by severe 'girdle' pains round her lower chest as the vertebral collapse impinges on the emerging nerve roots.

Diagnosis is by X-ray, for in uncomplicated cases the laboratory tests are remarkable for their normality. The normal ESR excludes myelomatosis as a cause of the vertebral collapse, while the normal (or near normal) serum alkaline phosphatase excludes other bone diseases such as osteomalacia, renal osteodystrophy, and Paget's disease of bone. However, secondary carcinoma is not excluded by a normal ESR and alkaline phosphatase, and secondary deposits from cancer of the female breast, male prostate, or lung have always to be considered.

In the gross case the spinal X-ray changes are highly characteristic. They are illustrated in Figure 9.2 and include:

1. Loss of bone density. This sign has to be interpreted with care. The safe rule is to regard it as positive only when the density of the central part of the vertebral bodies is as radiolucent as the inter-vertebral disc spaces.
2. 'Cod fish' vertebrae. The intervertebral disc becomes lens shaped, with the central part bulging into the vertebral bodies to give them a biconcave shape.

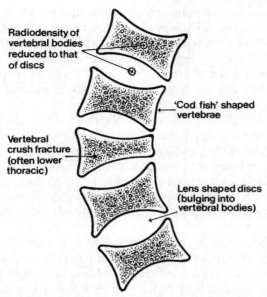

Radiodensity of
vertebral bodies
reduced to that
of discs

'Cod fish' shaped
vertebrae

Vertebral
crush fracture
(often lower
thoracic)

Lens shaped discs
(bulging into
vertebral bodies)

Fig. 9.2. Lateral view of osteoporotic spine. Diagram to illustrate radiological changes.

3. Crush fractures, often with 'wedging' of multiple vertebrae. The pattern of the crush is seldom helpful. It is the preservation of the intervertebral disc space which differentiates both osteoporosis and malignant deposits from infections (see Figure 8.1).

Management is not as hopeless as might be expected. These crush fractures do tend to heal. The initial painful stages require analgesia and restriction of back movements. However, like ankylosing spondylitis (p. 50) this is a condition in which rest is positively harmful and, as soon as possible, graded trunk exercises are started. The objective is to slow down the rate of mineral loss by the stimulus of muscle activity. A therapeutic pool is ideal for this, but the physiotherapist can also provide a 'dry land' exercise programme which is helpful.

Drug therapy aimed at increasing the bone mass is not dramatically effective. Some favour oestrogen supplements, vitamin D, calcitonin or fluoride, but all of these have potential drawbacks. Modest calcium supplementation is safe and is probably worth employing. A convenient preparation is Sandocal (Sandoz) a lactate–gluconate preparation given as a single dose of four effervescent tablets on retiring.

Osteomalacia

Vitamin D is necessary for the adequate mineralization of bones. Lack of the vitamin causes osteomalacia in adults and rickets in children. There are two sources of the vitamin: ingestion with food and synthesis in the skin. The former requires adequate absorption of fats (the vitamin is fat-soluble) and the latter requires adequate exposure of the skin to ultra-violet radiation. Lack of vitamin D usually results from a combination of factors, including inadequate diet, malabsorption, and lack of sunlight exposure.

In Britain the group most commonly affected by osteomalacia is Asian immigrants, particularly Gujarati vegan women, and the usual cause is a combination of inadequate dietary intake and lack of sunlight exposure, sometimes combined with repeated pregnancies. Similar factors may lead to osteomalacia in the elderly of any racial group, particularly those living alone. Occasionally steatorrhoea is a contributing cause, rarely it may result from interaction with chronically administered anticonvulsant drugs.

Unlike osteoporosis, the osteomalacic bones are spontaneously painful. They are tender to pressure and painful to move. The pains may mimic rheumatic disorders closely. Muscular weakness is another characteristic feature. Any Asian with this type of complaint should be suspected of osteomalacia. Fortunately the serum alkaline phosphatase concentration provides a convenient screening test. It is usually markedly elevated in any patient with osteomalacia, and the diagnosis is confirmed by low serum concentrations of vitamin D. In addition, in well-developed cases, the radiological appearance is often characteristic, with 'pseudo-fractures' of the bony rami of the pelvis or the upper femora. These translucent lines look like un-united and un-displaced fractures running transversely across the bones, and they are usually bilaterally symmetrical.

A blood urea or creatinine determination should be carried out to exclude the possibility that these appearances are due to renal osteodystrophy.

Straightforward osteomalacia due to lack of dietary vitamin D and sunlight deprivation is treated by giving the vitamin (calciferol) by mouth in a dose of 10 000 units (calciferol tablets, high-strength) three times a week.

Skeletal pains should resolve in about 4 weeks, but weakness may persist for a year. Patients with steatorrhea may require parenteral administration. Patients with renal failure or other rare renal causes of vitamin-D-resistant rickets may require much larger doses. These are best supervised by a specialized metabolic unit because of the danger of hypercalcaemia.

Hyperparathyroid bone disease

Overactivity of the parathyroid glands may be asymptomatic and discovered only because the serum calcium concentration is elevated on routine blood screening. It may also present with the symptoms of urinary calculi, or with pyrophosphate arthropathy (p. 73), or with metabolic bone disease. Like osteomalacia, this bone disease may be primary, or secondary to chronic renal failure. Renal osteodystrophy represents the combination of the bone changes of osteomalacia and hyperparathyroidism.

This type of metabolic bone disease may be asymptomatic, or may present with bone pain and tenderness, or fractures. The laboratory features are a raised serum calcium (over 2.60 mmol/l on repeated testing of fasting specimens obtained without venous stasis), and an elevated serum alkaline phosphatase. Cases with renal failure will also show evidence of this. Raised serum parathyroid hormone concentrations may provide confirmation. X-rays may be highly characteristic with fine sub-periosteal erosions of the terminal phalanges of the fingers. Severe cases may show gross distortion of trabecular patterns and localized cystic 'brown tumours', chondrocalcinosis and even fractures.

Treatment is directed at the primary defect (parathyroid gland or kidney), but vitamin D may be used in an attempt to reduce any element of osteomalacia.

Paget's disease of bone

Paget's disease is not primarily a metabolic disorder of bone. It is very common, but the aetiology is unknown. Part or whole of single or multiple bones may be affected, usually in older patients. Pathologically there is excessive turnover of bone leading to a disordered trabecular structure. The lesions are highly vascular.

Paget's disease is usually asymptomatic and discovered by chance on X-ray or by finding a high concentration of serum alkaline phosphatase on routine biochemical screening. The most common mechanism of pain is involvement of a joint surface (e.g. hip or shoulder) leading to secondary osteoarthritis. Rarely, gross softening and bowing of bones may lead to severe, intractable bone pain.

Clinically there may be visible bowing of the affected bones (e.g. the tibia) and overlying warmth and tenderness. Rarely, very extensive involvement may produce features of high cardiac output through the increased vascularity. Since the affected bones enlarge the cranial nerves may become trapped as they leave the skull producing, e.g. deafness. Very rarely a sarcomatous change supervenes.

Laboratory tests reveal a high concentration of serum alkaline phosphatase (even with quite small and localized lesions) and a normal serum calcium concentration (unless the patient has been immobilized in bed, when it may be elevated). X-rays generally show the highly characteristic widening of affected segments of bones, together with gross coarsening of the trabecular pattern. Involved joints show the features of secondary osteoarthritis.

Most patients with Paget's disease of bone require no treatment (unless it be for secondary osteoarthritis). For those with spontaneous bone pain a variety of forms of treatment are available, all of which act by suppressing the rate of bone turnover. These include intramuscular calcitonin injections, various oral diphosphonate compounds, and the antimetabolite mithramycin. This is at present an experimental and changing area of therapy, and management is probably best undertaken in conjunction with a unit specializing in metabolic bone diseases.

HYPERTROPHIC OSTEOARTHROPATHY

The mechanism by which patients with conditions such as bronchial carcinoma or bronchiectasis develop finger clubbing is unknown. It is clear, however, that severe clubbing—whatever the underlying cause—is occasionally associated with a troublesome arthritis of the extremities. This is sometimes an early feature, and carcinoma of the bronchus can present with a complaint of arthritis.

The patient generally complains of a diffuse 'bursting' pain in the hands, sometimes in the feet, which is worse when the extremities are warmed under the bedclothes at night. Examination reveals hands which are somewhat puffy and tender over the small joints, but the range of movement is reasonably full. Finger clubbing is usually severe.

The diagnosis of osteoarthropathy is established by X-ray: films of the extremities show a fine, fuzzy line of periosteal new bone formation around the lower ends of the shafts of the humerus, radius, tibia, and fibula, and sometimes around the small bones of the hands and feet. The association is most often with a bronchial carcinoma, but osteo-arthropathy may occur with severe finger clubbing from any cause, including cyanotic heart disease.

Treatment is symptomatic. Anything which corrects the underlying cause, however, will relieve the arthropathy and, for reasons which are not clear, resecting a bronchial neoplasm, or even section of the vagus nerve on the affected side, may provide dramatic relief.

NEUROPATHIC (CHARCOT'S) JOINTS

Conditions which damage the sensory nerve supply from a joint tend to cause a gross, destructive (but painless), type of arthropathy. The exact mechanism is not clear. It may be that the loss of pain sensation removes a normal mechanism of warning about what may damage the joint, and this makes the joint more vulnerable. The pathological changes are those of very gross osteoarthritis.

A variety of conditions may cause Charcot joints. The traditional ones are tabes dorsalis (affecting the lower limbs) and syringomyelia (affecting the hands). However, anything which interferes with the afferent nerve supply from a joint may be responsible (e.g. diabetic neuropathy).

The condition is rare and the diagnosis easily missed. The patient is likely to complain of swelling, deformity, and disability, rather than pain, and examination reveals a joint which is often grossly swollen, unstable, grates loudly on passive movement, but is quite painless. X-rays confirm the gross destructive changes with new bone formation and loose bodies. Once the condition is suspected the sensory loss is usually easily detected. Tabetic cases typically have Argyll Robertson pupils and absent tendon reflexes, while 'dissociated anaesthesia' in the arms is the hallmark of syringomyelia. Diabetic neuropathy may occasionally be painful in the small joints of the foot.

Treatment aims at protecting the joint from trauma. This may involve the use of splints and walking aids, and the restriction of activities. There is doubt about whether these joints are suitable for arthroplasty.

SARCOIDOSIS

Sarcoidosis is an inflammatory multi-system disease of unknown aetiology. The characteristic histological lesion is an epitheliod-cell granuloma which somewhat resembles a tuberculous granuloma, except that caseation does not occur, and tubercle bacilli are absent. These patients tend to show altered immunological reactivity, with a reduced cell-mediated response to antigens such as tuberculin. Almost any system may be involved, the most common being lungs, lymph nodes, eyes, and skin.

Arthritis occurs in sarcoidosis in two different circumstances. The more serious form is that in which the joints are involved together with other systems such as the lungs, skin, eyes, salivary glands, and bones, and the features are those of a chronic destructive arthritis affecting one or a few joints. This form may be mistaken for rheumatoid arthritis, but histology reveals the typical granulomata. In Britain this pattern of arthritis is rare except amongst West Indian immigrants. Management of this multi-system sarcoidosis is not modified because of the joint involvement.

The benign form is more common in Britain. It affects young adults, particularly women, and does not show a predilection for immigrants. The typical history is for a previously fit young woman to present with erythema nodosum (see above), fever and arthritis of one or a few lower-limb joints. Chest X-rays reveal bilateral hilar lymph-node enlargement.

The prognosis for complete recovery is excellent, and the arthritis resolves uneventfully over a few weeks or, at most, months. This appears to be a benign variety of sarcoidosis, and is referred to as Lofgren's syndrome. Progression from this to more generalized, granulomatous sarcoidosis has been described, but is rare. Only symptomatic treatment is required, but if the arthritis is very troublesome it may be justifiable to give a limited course of corticosteroids.

SERUM SICKNESS (IMMUNE-COMPLEX DISEASE)

In the earlier part of the present century, before antibiotics were available, the main weapon for treating many established bacterial infections (e.g. diphtheria) was passive immunization with serum from horses rendered immune to bacteria or their toxins. A major drawback to this form of therapy was the frequent occurrence of serum sickness. About 10 days after the injection the patient would develop fever, urticaria, proteinuria, and polyarthritis. It is now known that this was due to the formation of circulating immune complexes. The sequence of events is illustrated in Figure 9.3. The large dose of foreign protein (horse serum) evokes an antibody response in the patient. This helps to remove the foreign protein but, when the ratio of antigen to antibody reaches a critical point of slight antigen excess, soluble immune complexes tend to be deposited in the lining of the blood vessels, leading to inflammation. Fixation of complement and attraction of neutrophils

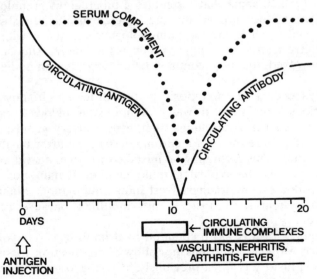

Fig. 9.3. Diagram illustrating the sequence of immunological events in serum sickness.

are essential steps in the inflammation. The consumption of complement is reflected in lowered levels of complement components in the serum (Fig. 9.3).

Serum therapy is hardly ever used nowadays. However, a similar pattern of illness occurs in a variety of circumstances. Examples are the systemic reaction which may occasionally follow the administration of drugs such as penicillin, or the transient polyarthritis which may occur during the early phase of hepatitis (p. 108). These reactions are recognized as being due to immune-complex formation by the clinical association of fever, urticarial skin eruptions, proteinuria, and polyarthritis. A variety of laboratory tests can be used to identify immune complexes in the circulation (see Appendix 1). For convenience the term serum sickness continues to be used to describe this clinical reaction pattern. It implies a disease caused by circulating immune complexes. This is usually a transient phenomonon. If the offending antigen is not removed, however, chronic renal disease or fatal vasculitis may result. Transient lowering of serum complement components is probably the most useful laboratory marker of immune complex disease (Fig. 9.3 and Appendix 1).

At a practical level, when the clinical picture of serum sickness (e.g. urticaria and arthritis) is encountered, it is necessary to consider whether the cause may be a drug, and to exclude the possibility of an early hepatitis virus infection.

REFERENCES

Ansell, B. M. (1970). Henoch–Schönlein purpura with particular reference to the prognosis of the renal lesion. *Br. J. Dermatol.* **82**, 211–15.

Barnes, C. G. and Colvin, B. T. (1983). Haemophilia. In *Reports on Rheumatic Diseases: Collected Reports 1959–1983,* pp. 64–8. Arthritis and Rheumatism Council, London.

Biggs, R. (ed.) (1978). *The treatment of haemophilia A and B and von Willebrand's disease.* Blackwells, Oxford.

Bird, H. A., Tribe, C. R., and Bacon, P. A. (1978). Joint hypermobility leading to osteoarthritis and chondrocalcinosis. *Ann. Rheum. Dis.* **37**, 203–11.

Blomgren, S. E. (1974). Erythema nodosum. *Seminars in arthritis and rheumatism.* (ed. Talbot, J. H.). **4**, 1–24. Grune and Stratton, New York.

Brower, A. C. and Allman, R. M. (1981). The neuropathic joint: a neurovascular bone disorder. *Radiol. Clin. North America* **19**, 571–80.

Cohen, R. D. (1986). Metabolic bone disease. In *Mason and Currey's Clinical rheumatology.* Currey, H. L. F. (ed) (4th edn). Pitman Medical, London.

Fitzgerald, A. A. and Davis, P. (1982). Arthritis, hilar adenopathy, erythema nodosum complex. *J. Rheumatol.* **9**, 935–8.

O'Duffy, J. D., Lehner, T., and Barnes, C. G. (1983). Summary of the third international conference on Behçet's disease. *J. Rheumatol.* **10**, 154–8.

Schneerson, J. M. (1981). Digital clubbing and hypertrophic osteoarthropathy: the underlying mechanisms. *Br. J. Dis Chest* **75**, 113–31.

Schumacher, H. R. (1975). Rheumatological manifestations of sickle cell disease and other haemoglobinopathies. *Clinics in rheumatic diseases.* (ed Berger, P. E. and Kulen, J. P.) **1**, 37–52. W. B. Saunders, London.

Steven, M. M., Yogarajah, S., Madhok, R., Forbers, C. D., and Sturrock, R. D. (1986). Haemophilic arthritis. *Quart. J. Med.* **58**, 181–97.

Truelove, L. H. (1960). Articular manifestations of erythema nodosum. *Ann. Rheum. Dis.* **19**, 174–80.

Vaughan, J. H., Barnett, E. V., and Leadley, P. (1967). Serum sickness: evidence in man of antigen–antibody complexes and free light chains in the circulation during the acute reaction. *Ann. Int. Med.* **67**, 301–15.

Yurdakul, S., Yazici, H., Tuzun, Y., *et al.* (1983). The arthritis of Behçet's disease. *Ann. Rheum. Dis.* **42**, 505–15.

10 Regional problems I:

The neck

Disorders of the neck are common in general practice, second only in incidence to disorders of the lumbar spine. The majority are caused by mechanical lesions of the cervical vertebrae and surrounding structures. A small minority of disorders cause pressure damage to the cervical portion of the spinal cord, calling for urgent assessment and specialist attention. The remainder are caused by tumours and other conditions.

Incidence of neck problems in General Practice

In 1977 Billings and Mole analysed 1000 consecutive patients seen in general practice with a new presenting complaint. 10.6 per cent had a rheumatological problem, and a classification by anatomical region of the body produced the figures shown in Table 10.1.

Table 10.1. *Incidence of rheumatological problems by anatomical region affected (from Billings and Mole 1977).*

Neck	15	Temporomandibular joint	2
Thoracic	5	Elbow	3
Shoulder	8	Wrist	6
Lumbar spine	29	Knee	8
Hip	4	Ankle	5
Hand	8	Foot	6
General symptoms	7		
Total number of patients: 106			

CERVICAL SPONDYLOSIS AND ACUTE CERVICAL DISC LESIONS

The term cervical spondylosis is used to describe degenerative changes affecting the intervertebral discs of the neck (Fig. 10.1). A term distinct from osteoarthritis is necessary because the disc joints are non-synovial. However, osteoarthritis can affect the posterior facet (apophyseal) joints of the cervical spine which are small synovial articulations (see Chapter 2).

The intervertebral disc is composed of a spongy central core, the nucleus pulposus, and a fibrous outer rim, the annulus fibrosus. This is

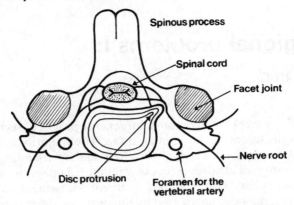

Fig. 10.1. A segment of the cervical spine showing the nerve root, a disc protrusion, the facet joint, and the foramen surrounding the vertebral artery.

thickened at the back and front to form the anterior and posterior longitudinal ligaments. The discs are able to absorb enormous stress, but over the course of time degenerative damage is extremely common. Disc substance or fragments can herniate vertically into the vertebra above or below, producing Schmorl's nodes (Fig. 2.11) which can be seen clearly on X-rays (at autopsy as many as 40 per cent of spines show evidence of this condition), or horizontally through the annulus fibrosus. The commonest protrusions of clinical significance are postero-lateral, where they can encroach on the intervertebral foramen and press on the emerging nerve root (see Fig. 10.1). Lateral protrusions can also impinge on the vertebral arteries which pass up the cervical spine enclosed in their bony foramen. This may cause symptoms of vertebrobasilar insufficiency (p. 130). A disc protrusion will strip the periosteum from the bone surface and, in time, osteophyte formation will follow. A large osteophyte can encroach on the intervertebral foramen causing pressure on the nerve root and, occasionally, on the spinal cord. The apophyseal joints, being synovial, are prone to the development of osteoarthritis, and osteophytes from this site can also encroach on the emerging nerve root in the foramen.

Owing to the strength of the posterior longitudinal ligament a central, posterior disc herniation is very rare. Although rare it is of special significance as the disc fragments may cause direct pressure on the spinal cord, or, by pressure on the anterior spinal artery, ischaemic changes in the cord. Surgical decompression may then be necessary to prevent a quadriparesis.

In clinical practice, the nomenclature of the various syndromes associated with mechanical derangement of the spine can be confusing. This reflects the fact that it is very difficult to be certain which structures—whether bones, joints, discs, or ligaments—are actually the cause of the problem. A further difficulty is that standard radiography correlates very poorly with clinical symptoms, a spine showing gross evidence of cervical spondylosis may be completely symptom free, and vice versa. The authors support the term 'acute cervical disc lesion' for an acute episode of neck pain often associated with trauma, and the term 'cervical spondylosis' for a more chronic condition; characteristically with X-ray changes. However, many clinical syndromes fall part way between these extremes.

As might be expected for a condition which is largely caused by degenerative changes, the peak incidence is in late middle age, and affects the sexes equally (see Table 10.2).

Table 10.2. *Age-related incidence of cervical joint disorders*

Age of patient	Rate of cervical spondylosis per 1000 population
5–14	0.2
15–24	1.1
25–44	6.1
45–64	15.3
65–74	16.8
75 and over	12.5

Nerve root lesions and referred pain

The segments of the cervical spine correspond to the segmentation of the embryo. Damage to any of the structures which are derived from a particular segment may give rise to pain throughout the associated dermatome. A common observation is that the more severe the pain the more widely it is distributed throughout the dermatome. Hence damage to articular structures, ligaments, and the dural sheath of the nerve root will all cause pain throughout the dermatome, it follows from this that pain in a limb does not necessarily mean pressure on the nerve root. Reliable evidence of pressure on the nerve root itself includes parasthesiae, numbness and weakness of the muscles supplied by that root.

Table 10.3 shows a simplified list of the weaknesses and sensory changes associated with each nerve root. These are compared with the motor and sensory distribution of the three major peripheral nerves in the arm.

Figure 10.2 shows the distribution of the cutaneous dermatomes in the upper limb. These overlap extensively, hence sensory changes confined to one root are difficult to demonstrate objectively.

Table 10.3. *Comparative data on root and nerve lesions in the upper limb*

	Sensory loss	Motor deficit
C$_5$	Deltoid region	Supraspinatus Shoulder abduction Biceps Biceps reflex
C$_6$	Radial side of forearm thumb and index finger	Biceps Brachioradialis Supinator reflex
C$_7$	Dorsum of forearm middle finger	Triceps, wrist extensors Triceps jerk
C$_8$	Ulnar border of forearm 4th and 5th fingers	Finger flexors and extensors Thenar muscles in some patients
T$_1$	Ulnar border of arm and forearm	All small hand muscles, interossei and lumbricals
Radial nerve C$_{5,6,7}$	Back of hand between thumb and index finger	Triceps and brachioradialis Wrist and finger extension
Median nerve C$_{6,7,8}$T$_1$	Thumb, index, middle, and part of ring finger	Flexor carpi radialis Abductor pollicis brevis Oppenens pollicis
Ulnar nerve C$_8$T$_1$	Part of ring finger and 5th finger	Flexor carpi ulnaris interossei — adduction and abduction of fingers Adductor pollicis Ulnar 2 lumbricals (claw hand)

The whiplash injury

This is often understood by patients to be a condition with a specific form of treatment. In fact it only describes how a neck injury occurs. The commonest event is when a stationary vehicle is rammed from the rear; the unbraced neck undergoes acute extension followed by flexion. A severe whiplash injury can rupture the anterior longitudinal ligament and cause damage to the spinal cord. A moderate injury will cause a bout of cervical joint pain and pressure on the nerve root which may last for months. A minor injury will cause pain and stiffness which settles over a week or two. Treatment will depend on the symptoms, but in general is the same as for an acute disc lesion or cervical spondylosis.

Clinical presentation

There are various syndromes of mechanical joint lesions of the neck which will be familiar to GPs.

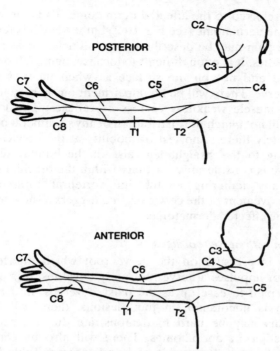

Fig. 10.2. The distribution of the cutaneous dermatomes in the upper limb. The dermatomes overlap, hence sensory changes confined to one root are difficult to demonstrate objectively.

Cervical pain with no symptoms or signs of nerve root involvement

Most people will have experienced a mild form of this as a 'cricked neck'. In children cervical pain and torticollis is often due to enlarged cervical lymph nodes, and will settle when the underlying condition resolves.

The history will not reliably distinguish between an acute disc lesion and cervical spondylosis. There may be a history of a jolt, such as in a whiplash injury, but often there is no obvious traumatic incident. The patient reports pain; this may spread from the occiput to the upper thoracic region, and laterally as far as the point of the shoulder. The six neck movements, flexion, extension, right and left rotation, and side flexion may be painful or restricted in range when compared to the opposite movement. The articular signs do not help to determine the exact level of the lesion, neither will local palpation: although extreme local tenderness would suggest more sinister pathology, such as an infection or a secondary deposit (see p. 134).

Cervical pain with nerve root symptoms

When a disc fragment or an oseophyte impinges on the dural covering to the nerve root, in addition to pain from the articular derangement, there will be pain referred to the affected dermatome. The pain may be felt in any part of the dermatome (see Fig. 10.2) but usually it is felt in the distal portion. The pain may be described as a dull ache, or as a sensation of pins-and-needles. It is often difficult to localize, being felt deep inside the arm or hand and not on the surface as when there is damage to a peripheral nerve. There will be no impairment on sensory testing, and no evidence of muscle weakness or loss or reflexes. The localization of symptoms will not match the distribution of any peripheral nerve.

Unfortunately there is no test of mobility at the cervical nerve roots corresponding to the straight leg raise in the lumbar region. This is because there is considerable elasticity within the brachial plexus, which will mask any tethering at the intervertebral foramen. However, sometimes movement of the cervical spine triggers a shower of 'pins-and-needles' in the affected dermatome.

Cervical pain with nerve root signs

When there is pressure on the nerve root which interferes with the conduction of impulses a nerve root palsy develops. It is quite common for the arm pain to ease up as the palsy develops. In a complete root palsy, which is uncommon in joint lesions, there will be cutaneous analgesia; this may be hard to demonstrate due to the considerable overlap of adjacent dermatomes. There will also be some degree of muscular weakness and alteration of the reflexes (see Table 10.3).

On occasion it may be difficult to distinguish a root lesion from a peripheral nerve disorder. Table 10.3 lists the main points of difference. If doubt remains electromyography will be helpful, and may suggest other uncomon conditions which at times mimic a nerve root lesion, such as motor neurone disease, syringomyelia, neuralgic amyotrophy and peripheral neuropathies.

Pressure on the spinal cord

A central disc protrusion can press on the spinal cord itself. Although this is very infrequent, it is one of the commonest causes of cervical cord compression in elderly people. It may occur suddenly (e.g. following a severe whiplash injury), but usually develops slowly and painlessly. Sometimes the patient will report tingling in the hands and feet brought on by flexion of the neck. As pressure on the cord gradually increases the patient will begin to notice difficulty with walking, and with bladder control. By this time long tract signs, including extensor plantar responses, should be obvious. A paraplegia may develop, often following pressure on the anterior spinal artery, causing ischaemia of the cord.

Vertebro-basilar artery insufficiency

The vertebral arteries pass up the neck partially enclosed by the foramina of the upper six cervical vertebrae. If the circle of Willis is interrupted due to atheromatous change, pressure on the vertebral artery will cause symptoms due to ischaemia of the cerebellum and occipital lobes. The common symptom, among the elderly, of vertigo on looking upwards is a mild manifestation. Other symptoms include vertigo on neck rotation, blurring of vision on sudden movements, or 'drop attacks'.

Differential diagnosis of the acutely painful neck

Although in general practice the most common cause of neck disorder is a mechanical lesion there is a wide differential to be considered:

1. Mechanical disorders of the cervical joint.
2. Muscular tension headaches.
3. Trauma and fractures.
4. Osteoporotic crush fractures.
5. Metastatic deposits.
6. Ankylosing spondylitis.
7. Neuralgic amyotrophy.
8. Polymyalgia and cranial arteritis.
9. Rheumatoid arthritis affecting the upper cervical spine.
10. Thoracic outlet syndromes.
11. Primary tumours, e.g. neurofibroma.

Management of mechanical disorders of the cervical joint

The great majority of patients seen in general practice with mechanical joint disease of the neck have cervical pain alone. A few will have symptoms of root pressure and a tiny minority will have damage to a nerve root.

The natural history of cervical pain of mechanical origin is that the majority of cases will settle spontaneously whatever treatment regimen is instituted. In general, neck pain on its own settles over a period of several weeks; if there is pressure on a nerve root, pain in the arm may be severe for several months. If a nerve root palsy develops one can predict that the limb pain will settle quickly, (although the neck pain may persist). Patients can be reassured that they will regain full power following a root palsy; this is because of peripheral neuronal sprouting from the nerve roots above and below the lesion, which will re-innervate the muscle fibres supplied by the damaged nerve root. Full power returns about six months after the palsy develops; the reflexes may be permanently altered.

All treatment regimens have to be compared with this tendency towards natural resolution. Active management might include the following:

Explanation

This is probably the most important aspect of treatment. If a patient understands the cause of the condition, the likely time it will take to resolve, and what can be done to help, he may well tolerate the pain better and be less likely to go on a fruitless search for an instant cure.

Temporary symptomatic relief

Temporary relief can be obtained from the application of heat, massage, counter irritants, and analgesic or non-steroidal anti-inflammatory drugs. Attention to posture, the use of a 'butterfly' pillow at night, and stopping people from putting their necks through a punishing exercise routine are all helpful.

A well-fitting cervical collar

A collar provides local heat, and reminds patients not to move their necks. There is no evidence that a particular type of collar is better than any other, so the most important criterion is acceptability to the patient.

Physiotherapy

Although these patients are frequently referred to physiotherapy departments exercises have not proved helpful, and local heat can be applied just as well by the patient at home with a hot water bottle. Cervical traction and manipulation of the neck are used in some departments. There is no doubt that some patients benefit from these measures, although they have never been adequately tested in a controlled trial. It is often difficult to separate the enormous psychological benefits of sympathetic attention from the supposed physical effects of the treatment regimen. Manipulation of the neck should not be undertaken unless X-rays have excluded any contraindications (rheumatoid, trauma, infection, osteoporotic collapse, multiple osteophytes).

Alternative medicine

Many patients attend osteopaths and other practitioners of 'alternative' medicine. Undoubtedly some patients are helped by a number of quite diverse treatments. The subject is discussed further in Chapter 17.

Standard X-rays

Standard X-rays are usually unhelpful unless there are severe osteophytic changes showing encroachment on the foramen. Many patients with gross X-ray changes are symptom free, and conversely a patient may have a severe cervical joint disorder with normal X-rays (although myelography or CT scanning may demonstrate a disc protrusion). It follows that standard radiography is used in the management of mechanical joint lesions for the following reasons:

To exclude other diseases such as metastases, infection or inflammatory joint disease.

To establish whether mobilization techniques can be used safely (see
above).

To reassure the patient.

Myelography is only indicated if surgical removal of a disc is considered,
or if the diagnosis is uncertain and an intraspinal tumour is a possibility.

Surgical decompression

Decompression is only indicated if pain is intractable, if there is evidence
of myelopathy, or if the diagnosis is in doubt.

OTHER CONDITIONS OF THE NECK

Thoracic outlet syndrome

The brachial plexus and the subclavian vessels pass through the
restricted space formed by the clavicle, the first rib and scalenus
anterior (see Fig. 10.3). If this space becomes constricted there will be
clinical evidence of pressure on the structures passing through it.
Symptoms are most frequently detected in the lower trunks of the
brachial plexus and the subclavian artery.

Causes of the thoracic outlet syndrome

Cervical ribs or fibrous bands

Many individuals have X-ray evidence of a cervical rib, but remain

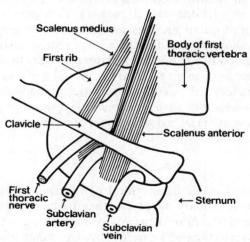

Fig. 10.3. The anatomy of the thoracic outlet.

completely symptom free. If symptoms develop they are frequently vascular, with a white, cold hand; sometimes there is evidence of a C_8, T_1 root palsy with wasting and weakness of the small muscles of the hand. Treatment is surgical.

Shoulder girdle droop

This is a cause of muscle wasting in the hands of the elderly patient. It occurs insidiously, and commonly the patient will complain of nocturnal pins-and-needles. This is a release phenomenon occurring as the brachial plexus is lifted off the first rib when the patient lies down for the night. Owing to the combination of nocturnal paraesthesiae and wasting in the hands it has to be distinguished from the carpal tunnel syndrome (p. 172), and is often difficult to distinguish from a C_7 disc lesion. Shoulder-raising exercises and avoiding heavy shopping bags may help the symptoms.

Pancoast's tumour

An apical lung carcinoma may erode the first two ribs, infiltrate the lower roots of the brachial plexus, and the sympathetic chain. Horner's syndrome and paralysis of C_8 and T_1 should always trigger a request for X-rays showing apical views of the lung.

Neuralgic amyotrophy (acute brachial neuritis)

The cause of this condition is unknown, it may on occasion follow a virus infection. There is acute onset of severe pain in the neck which spreads into the arm in the distribution of several nerve roots. (This condition also occurs in the lumbar–sacral plexus.) The pain is followed by paralysis of the appropriate muscles, and a variable sensory loss. Electromyography will show axonal damage with a patchy distribution across several roots. The pain may take two or three months to settle, and there is frequently some permanent residual loss of power. There is no specific treatment; the patient will need symptomatic management for the pain, which is often severe, and advice on exercises from a physiotherapist in an attempt to prevent the later development of a frozen shoulder.

Spinal tumours

Secondary deposits occur at any level of the spine. Unless there is a history of a known primary neoplasm, they frequently go unrecognized for some time under a false diagnosis of mechanical joint lesion. This underlines the importance of a careful physical examination, looking for evidence of the commoner malignancies such as breast, lung and prostate. Points which should suggest a search for evidence of malignant deposits include:

Rapidly increasing severe pain.
Unremitting pain at rest.
Local tenderness.
Neurological signs at more than one root level. (This does not occur in cervical spondylosis because the nerve roots emerge in a horizontal position.)
C_8 or T_1 paresis, rarely caused by mechanical joint lesions.

X-rays, a raised ESR and alkaline phosphatase, and a bone scan will aid the diagnosis. An expanding metastasis will cause a dense root paresis (unlike cervical spondylosis) and may cause cord pressure with long tract signs. Symptomatic treatment with radiotherapy may give considerable pain relief and so early referral is important.

The commonest primary tumours are myeloma and the benign neurofibroma. Myeloma may cause vertebral crush fractures or an expanding bone lesion producing symptoms similar to secondary deposits. Neurofibromata can develop in the intervertebral foramina causing considerable pain and a progressive root paresis. Root pain which persists and gets worse over several months is a common history. Oblique views of the cervical spine may show an expanded foramen; treatment is surgical.

REFERENCES

Billings, R. A. and Mole, K. F. (1977). Rheumatology in General Practice: a survey in world rheumatism year. *J. R. Coll. Gen. Pract.* **27**, 721–5.
Cyriax, J. (1982). *Textbook of orthopaedic medicine.* Vol. 1 (8th edn). Balliere Tindall, London.

11 Regional problems II:

The lower back

Low back pain ranks with upper respiratory tract infection as one of the most common conditions seen in general practice. As with respiratory infection, it is a heterogenous condition and there is as yet no clear consensus on the management of the different syndromes. In recent years there has been considerable research into the natural history, the prognostic features, and the value of certain treatments, so clearer guidance may emerge in the future.

The office of Health Economics reported that in 1984 there were two million consultations with GPs for back trouble. Some 63 000 people were admitted to hospital for a stay averaging 12 days. The cost to the nation is high, annually 33 million working days are lost, which is about 10 per cent of all certified sick leave. When translated into the statistics of an average practice this means that about 3 per cent of adult patients consult their doctor annually about low back pain. In Billings and Mole's general practice survey of 1000 consecutive patients with a new presenting complaint (see Table 10.1 Chapter 10), one in ten had a rheumatological problem, and of these 30 per cent had low back pain. By far the commonest cause of low back pain in general practice is damage to the discs and joints, but other important causes should not be ignored (Table 11.1). Frequently their initial presentation is indistinguishable from pain of mechanical origin, and only regular review over time can distinguish them.

Functional anatomy of the spine

As in the cervical spine the lumbar vertebrae are separated by spongy discs and bound together by ligaments. The strong paraspinal muscles, sacrospinalis and iliopsoas, are extensors and flexors of the spine respectively.

The main differences in anatomy from the cervical spine are as follows:

The nerve roots emerge obliquely, rather than horizontally, so that it is possible for a prolapsed disc to cause pressure on more than one nerve root. The spinal cord ends at the level of L_1, hence a large central protrusion below L_1 will cause pressure on the cauda equina (resulting in saddle or peri-anal sensory changes), but there will be no long tract signs. Owing to the shape of the spine a prolapsed disc is most likely to cause

Table 11.1.   *Causes of low back pain*

Mechanical back pain	Disc lesions
	Spondylosis
	Muscle and ligament lesions
Structural disorders	Spondylolisthesis
	Fractures
	Spinal stenosis
Inflammatory lesions	Ankylosing spondylitis
	Other B27-related conditions
Metabolic disorders	Osteoporosis
	Osteomalacia
	Paget's disease
Infections	Tuberculosis
	Osteomyelitis
Neoplasms	Primary, e.g. myeloma
	neurofibromata
	retroperitoneal
	masses
	Secondaries, e.g. breast
	prostate
	lung
Psychogenic	Aches and pains may be the presenting complaint in a depressed or anxious patient

nerve root pressure at L_5 and S_1, and least likely to cause neurological signs at L_1 and L_2 (Fig. 11.1).

The lower sacral vertebrae are fused at the sacrum and wedged between the iliac bones (Fig. 11.2). The sacro-iliac joints are synovial, but permit very little movement. They are frequently fused; this causes no clinical problem.

Examining the spine

The unclothed spine should be examined from the rear. Kyphosis and scoliosis should be noted (see p. 150), and the spinous processes of the vertebrae palpated for evidence of local tenderness.

Articular signs (signs relating to disordered joints)

The range of spinal movements varies considerably between individuals. It begins to decline at middle age when disc degeneration and osteophyte formation cause a physical block to the range of movement. Many spines that are almost rigid cause their owners no pain and little restriction of

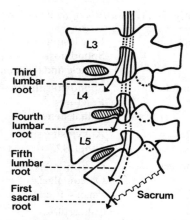

Fig. 11.1. A diagram of a segment of the lumbar spine, showing the site of a prolapse of the nucleus pulposus causing an L_5 nerve entrapment. Note that a disc protrusion at this level may compress more than one spinal nerve.

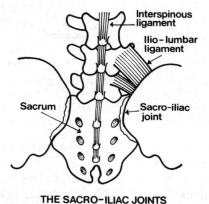

THE SACRO-ILIAC JOINTS

Fig. 11.2. The lower lumbar spine, sacrum and sacro-iliac joints.

their activities. Indeed, one school of thought suggests that the development of osteophytes is beneficial, providing a form of internal corset for the spine and preventing movements which might otherwise cause a disc prolapse. When examining the range of movement in a spine, the primary objective is to look for spasm in the lumbar muscles, for movements which trigger pain (such as flexion and extension in mechanical back pain), and for the stiff lumbar segment and restricted lateral flexion found in the spine with ankylosing spondylitis or other inflammatory arthritis.

Extension of the spine and forward flexion should be watched. Is the patient bending at the lumbar spine, or only at the hips? (Patients with ankylosing spondylitis may be able to get their hands on the floor if they have mobile hips.) Lateral flexion ('slide your hand down the side of your leg as far as it will go') should be examined for symmetry, and the patient asked to pinpoint the painful sites as they develop.

The hips should be examined (see p. 176): a diseased hip, or other leg joint, may cause pain in the lumbar spine. The sacro-iliac joints lie under the dimples of the upper buttock (Fig. 4.1), firm pressure at this site may elicit local tenderness. Firm pressure over the centre of the sacrum will also cause sacro-iliac pain (Fig. 4.2). Alternatively, the joints can be examined with the patient lying supine; the examiner's hands push down on the iliac crests attempting to open out the pelvic ring (Fig. 11.3). This manoeuvre will cause localized pain over an inflamed sacro-iliac joint.

Dural sheath pressure signs

The nerve roots are enclosed in a covering of dura mater. If there is a disc prolapse, the nerve roots may become tethered at the intervertebral foramen and anything which causes tension on the nerve roots or the dura mater will cause pain. Normally there is considerable elasticity at the sciatic plexus to allow for hip flexion.

Lying supine, the straight leg raise test (SLR) is performed (Fig. 11.4). This stretches the sciatic plexus ($L_{4,5}$, $S_{1,2}$). If the nerve roots are tethered, the hamstrings will go into spasm to protect the nerve roots from further damage, and the patient will report back or leg pain. Sometimes there is a crossed response, when elevation of the pain-free leg causes pain in the back and the affected leg. This does not necessarily mean that the protrusion is bilateral but simply that this movement is also causing tension on the opposite nerve root and dural sheath. The SLR test can be done in a variety of different positions (Fig. 11.4(a), (b), (c)), which may

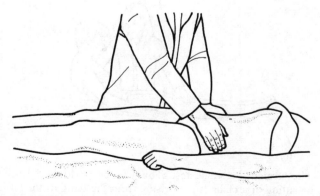

Fig. 11.3. Examining the sacro-iliac joints with the patient supine.

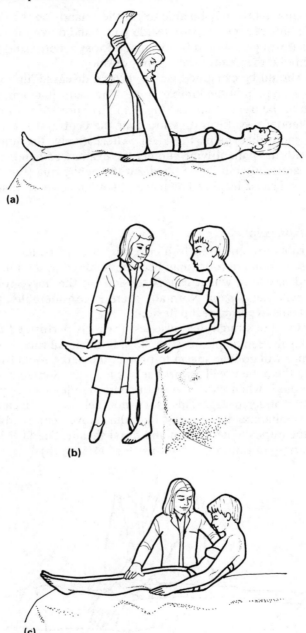

Fig. 11.4. The straight leg raise test. This can be performed with the patient supine (a), or sitting in a chair (b), or rising from the lying to the sitting position with straight legs (c).

help to separate out the psychological from the organic components of pain expressed by the patient.

Usually, with an acute prolapse, all three tests illustrated in Fig. 11.4 should give the same results. A discrepancy between the test in positions (a) and (c) suggests an exaggerated pain response. The femoral nerve stretch test is equivalent to the SLR for higher nerve roots. The patient lies prone, and the examiner passively flexes each knee in turn. If the L_3 root is tethered it will be painfully stretched by this procedure and pain will be felt in the anterior thigh and sometimes in the back. Sometimes crossed pain occurs as in the SLR. The test is not as unequivocal as the SLR, but is often of help in sorting out an uncharacteristic pain.

Further tests which suggest dural irritation include raising the head off the bed during the SLR; this stretches the dura from above. Coughing, straining, and sneezing raise the venous pressure and pull the dura upwards. These manouvres pull on the tethered nerve and cause pain.

Nerve root signs

Pressure damage to the nerve root causes pain which can spread throughout the corresponding dermatome (see Fig. 11.5). If the damage is severe, numbness and muscular weakness also develop. If the nerve root atrophies due to persistent pressure, the pain in the leg disappears

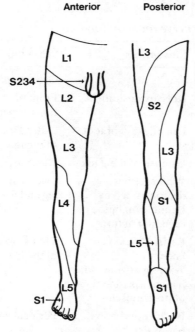

Fig. 11.5. The dermatomes of the lower limb.

and a total root palsy supervenes. The patient feels better although the anatomical situation has worsened. In general a disc prolapse only causes a partial paralysis, and a dense root lesion suggests more sinister pathology, particularly at the upper lumbar roots where mechanical lesions are rare. The nerve roots in the leg can be tested swiftly by choosing one muscle for every root. Table 11.2 sets out such a scheme. Table 11.3 compares root lesions with the common peripheral nerve lesions in the leg.

Experiments on volunteers have shown that irritation of many of the non-neural structures in the back such as ligaments, muscle and periosteum, can cause pain to be felt in any part of the developmental dermatome. Thus pain in the leg does not necessarily imply that there is pressure on the nerve root, and it is important to look for the positive signs of dural sheath pressure or nerve root signs before making this diagnosis.

As with damage to the cervical roots, patients can be reassured that damage to the muscles supplied by a single nerve root will recover fully. Peripheral neuronal sprouting from the nerve roots above and below the lesion will eventually re-innervate the muscles. However, it is not uncommon to get partial damage to two adjacent nerve roots, in which

Table 11.2. *Tests of nerve root conduction*

	Muscle	Movements	Sensation	Reflex
L_2	Psoas	Hip flexion	Groin to patella	None
L_3	Quadriceps	Knee extension	Front of thigh Inner aspect of leg	Knee jerk
L_4	Tibialis anterior	Dorsiflexion of foot	Outer aspect of thigh, shin and big toe	
L_5	Extensor hallucis	Extension of big toe	Outer aspect of leg	
S_1	Gastrocnemius	Weakness best demonstrated by standing on tiptoe on each foot in turn	Outer aspect of leg and foot	Ankle jerk
S_2	Hamstrings	Resisted flexion of knee	Thin strip down back of thigh and leg	None
	Glutei	Wasting obvious when patient asked to tighten buttock muscles		
$S_{3/4}$	Perineal muscles (Cauda equina)	Bladder and bowel paralysis	Perineal anaesthesia	None

Table 11.3. *Root lesion or peripheral nerve lesion in the leg*

Roots	Sensory loss	Motor deficit	Peripheral nerve	Sensory loss	Motor deficit
L_1 L_2	Front and lateral aspect of thigh	Rarely involved in disc lesions Hip flexion	Lateral cutaneous nerve of the thigh (common and often persistent)	Lateral thigh	none
L_3 L_4	Lower thigh Outer aspect of thigh and leg	Knee extension Dorsiflexion of foot			
L_5	Medial side of foot	Extension of big toe Inversion of foot	Common peroneal nerve usually damaged by pressure at the upper end of the fibula, causing foot drop	Lateral calf and dorsum of foot	Dorsiflexion of foot Dorsiflexion of toes Eversion of foot Ankle reflex normal
S_1	Outer aspect of leg, foot and sole	Gastrocnemius hamstrings Reduced ankle reflex	Tibial nerve compressed at the posterior aspect of tibia (rare)	Heel and sole of foot	Flexors of toes Intrinsic muscles of foot Soleus and gastrocnemius

case recovery of power may not be complete. If a reflex disappears it does not always return.

MECHANICAL LOW BACK PAIN

Nomenclature

Considerable confusion exists in the literature about the classification and terminology of mechanical causes of lumbar pain. Acute or chronic back strain, prolapsed disc, lumbago, sciatica, fibrositis, sprained sacro-iliac ligaments—these are a few of the more common terms used. The confused terminology reflects the fact that, for most patients with back pain encountered in general practice, a full history and a careful examination does not enable the doctor to identify which tissues are at fault. Moreover, the treatment given is largely empirical, and the effectiveness of many regularly used treatments (as well as the more heterodox procedures) is only just beginning to be rigorously tested. It must also be remembered that all treatments are strongly affected by the placebo response, and need to be assessed against the natural tendency to spontaneous improvement.

In this book the terms *acute* or *chronic low back pain* will be used, regardless of the pathogenic mechanisms, wherever there is mechanical low back pain without evidence of neurological involvement. *Prolapsed intervertebral disc* will be used whenever there is evidence of pressure on, or damage to, the nerve root. *Sciatica* will refer to nerve root pain extending down the side or back of the leg to the foot.

Epidemiology

Only a small proportion of people who experience back pain attend the doctor. A population survey from Ohio (Nagi, Riley, and Newby 1973) showed that 18 per cent of adults between 18 and 64 years of age are often bothered with pains in their backs. Women in all occupational groups were more likely to mention back pain than men, and men doing heavy manual work reported more than office workers. Two surveys of British general practice in the 1960s showed that between 2 and 3 per cent of the population over 15 years of age attend their doctors with back pain in the course of one year. Nearly half of these had a recurrence within four years.

As is to be expected of a mechanical degenerative condition there is a marked variation in age-related incidence for both men and women (see Table 11.4).

Table 11.4. *The age-related incidence of low back pain (from Ward, Knoweldon, and Sharrard 1968)*

Age	Rate per 1000 population male	Rate per 1000 population female
15–24	10.5	7.8
25–44	24.5	19.8
45–64	31.5	18.9
65+	14.3	7.6

Clinical presentation

Acute low back pain of mechanical origin usually presents in one of two ways.

(a) Sudden onset of low back pain often related to bending, twisting or lifting. The patient may be unable to straighten up, and the pain may extend down the buttocks to the thighs. There is usually considerable protective muscular spasm, restriction of most lumbar spine movements, and occasionally evidence of pressure on the nerve roots. This is often called 'lumbago' by the patient, and there may be recurrent attacks.

(b) Gradual onset of increasing back pain over several days. The patient is often concerned that what started as a mild ache in the lumbar region has spread over several days to become acute pain, sometimes with symptoms of nerve root involvement. The usual explanation for this progressive development of symptoms is the slow release of gelatinous disc contents through a tear in the annulus fibrosus.

Chronic low back pain is a frequent complaint in general practice. It is most common in the middle-aged; sometimes it is related to physical exertion, sometimes to the patient's emotional state, occasionally it is the presenting symptoms of a masked depression. General examination may not always be informative since at this age restriction of range is common. X-rays may show degenerative changes which are not necessarily related to the symptoms. Chronic back pain is a symptom which both doctor and patient find hard to bear. The patient tends to want a specific diagnosis which the doctor cannot give, and he may begin to feel an impostor if repeatedly told that all the X-rays and tests are normal. It is sometimes more productive to approach the management of pain as a separate issue from the question of 'what is wrong with my back?' (See Chapter 17.) There are some patients who would convert their distress into another set of symptoms if they did not present with back pain; in these cases the doctor and patient usually reach a modus vivendi in which the patient continues to have back symptoms but the doctor is not pressed into doing unnecessary investigations.

Less common clinical presentations

Extra-segmental referred pain

Pain from acute or chronic low back pain may spread up towards the scapulae, anteriorly to the abdomen and groins and down to the coccyx, buttocks, and thighs. The distribution of pain is of no help in localizing the lesion.

Root pain or paralysis

Unilateral root pain or palsy is helpful in diagnosis, by pointing to the level of root involved. Sometimes root pain occurs alone with no obvious preceding back pain. Examples of this are unexplained pain in the big and second toe resulting from L_5 root pressure, or S_1 involvement causing numbness of the outer foot and outer portion of the lower leg.

Cauda equina pressure

This occurs if a large central disc protrusion is pressing on the lower sacral nerve roots before they emerge from their exit foraminae. Sphincter disturbance, whether of retention or incontinence, and perineal anaesthesia are the key symptoms. If these are present the patient should be referred urgently for myelography and laminectomy in order to preserve sphincter function. In practice, the commonest cause of bladder retention in a patient with back pain is inhibition of function due to enforced recumbency in combination with pain or medication; this is usually solved if the patient can get into a warm bath.

Prediction of outcome

Ninety per cent of those with back pain presenting in general practice will get better with simple advice and analgesics over the course of two to four weeks. The skill of the doctor lies in identifying the patients who will need a more active approach. A recent study (Roland *et al.* 1983) has shown that GPs are not very good at predicting which patients will have a poor outcome. The study showed that a limitation of the SLR to less than 60 degrees at initial examination, and duration of pain of more than a week prior to the consultation were the best predictors of a prolonged episode of illness. A patient with a past history of back pain was more likely to have a recurrence, but past history was unhelpful in prognosticating about the current episode.

Even among those patients referred to a hospital rheumatology department, over 90 per cent of patients recover uneventfully over a period of about 3 months. Only 2 per cent of patients from this selected population proceeded to laminectomy.

Management

Acute episodes of low back pain will settle in less than 2 weeks in 50 per cent of cases. The GP with access to radiology and physiotherapy services can manage well over 90 per cent of cases satisfactorily in primary care. While waiting for natural resolution the patient can be helped by the following measures.

Explanation

The nature of the problem needs careful explanation. Many patients are worried that they have bad arthritis, or that they will become seriously crippled in the future. Reassurance needs to be given that this is essentially a benign condition and that no special investigations or treatment are needed during the first two or three weeks during which most backs settle.

If the patient has symptoms of nerve root pressure the prognosis should be more guarded. Many cases will settle within three months, the vast majority within a year; during this time either the disc shrinks or the nerve root atrophies. As the nerve root atrophies the pain settles, but the patient may notice the development of numbness and weakness. Complete return of power can be predicted unless there is evidence of multiple nerve root pressure. With appropriate information of this kind many patients are prepared to wait for spontaneous recovery.

Bed rest

If the mattress sags a board placed under it will improve lumbar support. Some patients are most comfortable lying on the floor.

Analgesia

In the early stages of a disc prolapse the patient may be in acute pain and unable to relax or sleep. A strong painkiller (such as dihydrocodeine) in combination with a muscle relaxant (such as diazepam) will often relieve pain and encourage strict bed rest. After a few days when this is stopped, most patients need no further medication other than aspirin or paracetamol. Many patients with chronic back pain are prescribed non-steroidal anti-inflammatory drugs, but there is no·reason why these should work any better than simple analgesics. The pain relieving properties of heat in the form of hot baths and hot water bottles should not be underestimated. Many patients 'rub in' something (e.g. methyl salicylate liniment, or white liniment) which acts as a counter irritant. As long as the patient is aware of the temporary nature of the relief obtained, the benefit of doing something positive should be encouraged.

If the back pain persists beyond two or three weeks and if root signs are present, there may be considerable pressure from the patient for active treatment rather than waiting for a spontaneous cure. At some stage in a case of persistent back pain it is sensible to check the ESR, and if indications exist to do a chest X-ray. The patient may expect to have X-rays taken of the lumbar spine and may be reassured by a normal result, however, the diagnostic yield from early, routine, lumbar spine X-rays (in the absence of specific indications) is almost negligible (Currey *et al.* 1978). Nevertheless, it is essential to maintain an open mind about the diagnosis, and regularly review the history and the examination, as some of the other causes of back pain (Table 11.1) are often indistinguishable from a mechanical lesion in their early stages.

Further treatment will depend both on the choice of the patient and on local provision.

Osteopathy and chiropractors

Many patients see osteopaths for manipulative treatment and some feel better after doing so. However, a recent trial comparing osteopathic manipulation with short-wave diathermy and placebo, showed equally significant improvements in all three groups, suggesting that the osteopathic treatment may not be as specific as is sometimes suggested. (See Gibson, Harkness *et al.* (1985) and Chapter 17 on management.)

Physiotherapy

This is often prescribed and may involve manipulative treatment, heat treatments, lumbar traction, or exercises. Some departments run a 'back life group' which teaches the patient how to lift, and how to look after his back and manage episodes of back pain. This approach has been shown to be effective in diminishing the amount of back pain experienced during pregnancy.

Back supports

Corsets vary from an elasticated surgical belt to a rigid plaster-of-Paris cast. Some patients with chronic pain gain relief from a corset. Their main value is in maintaining the lumbar lordosis and in reminding the patient not to attempt certain movements. There is no evidence that they have a place in managing the common self-limiting disorders of the spine.

General advice

Maintaining the lumbar lordosis is thought to put less stress on the posterior longitudinal ligament. In the position of lordosis any movement of the disc tends to be anterior, well out of the way of the nerve roots. Attention to the type of chair used, and posture during driving, and at work, need to be stressed. Techniques of relaxation, and regular exercise such as swimming, may also help the chronic back sufferer. An information sheet giving general advice and showing good and bad

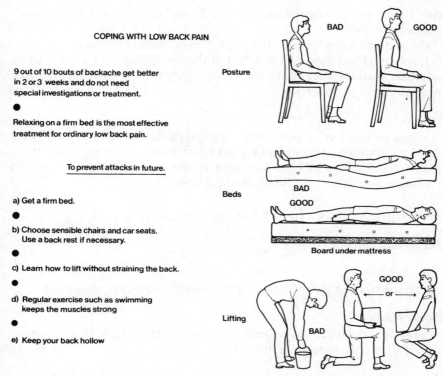

COPING WITH LOW BACK PAIN

9 out of 10 bouts of backache get better in 2 or 3 weeks and do not need special investigations or treatment.

Relaxing on a firm bed is the most effective treatment for ordinary low back pain.

To prevent attacks in future.

a) Get a firm bed.

b) Choose sensible chairs and car seats. Use a back rest if necessary.

c) Learn how to lift without straining the back.

d) Regular exercise such as swimming keeps the muscles strong

e) Keep your back hollow

Fig. 11.6. General advice on back care for patients with low back pain.

posture can be handed to the patient to underline the importance of self-management (see Fig. 11.6).

Further management options (available through departments of rheumatology or orthopaedics)

Epidural anaesthesia

Dilute local anaesthetic is instilled into the extra-dural space through the sacral hiatus. This often relieves the pain of sciatica dramatically for several hours; in some patients the effect is more long-lasting.

Surgery

Discectomy and removal of disc fragments is indicated in the following circumstances:

(a) Severe root pain that has been unresponsive to conservative measures, or has lasted more than a year. In this situation surgery is carried out to relieve pain; it usually relieves leg pain but has less effect on the back pain.

(b) Cauda equina lesions affecting bowel or bladder function.

(c) Extending neurological deficit. If there is evidence of a dense palsy affecting two adjacent roots the patient may be left with a noticeable weakness.

A pain clinic

A small minority of patients have chronic pain, maybe of several years standing, unrelieved by any of the previous treatment options. For these patients attention to the management of the pain rather than trying to eliminate the cause may provide the best help.

OTHER CAUSES OF MECHANICAL BACK PAIN

Structural defects

Spondylolysis

A congenital defect in the neural arch. In itself it causes no symptoms.

Spina bifida occulta

A posterior defect in the neural arch which is present in 20 per cent of spines. It has no clinical significance.

Spondylolisthesis

In this condition, which may be congenital or traumatic, there is forward slippage of the body of a lower lumbar vertebra in relationship to the vertebra below it. The condition is frequently symptomless, and may be a routine finding on X-ray. (About 5 per cent of pain free backs show this anomaly.) The unstable joint may cause an associated disc lesion, and occasionally results in persistent recurrent back pain. Treament is as for the disc lesion; surgery is indicated if there are signs of cauda equina pressure, if there is persistent pain, or rarely for instability.

Spinal stenosis

In this condition a congenitally narrow spinal canal will be further narrowed in middle life by bulging discs and bony osteophytes. The patient reports bilateral pain and numbness or weakness in the legs brought on by exercise. There are usually no positive findings on examination unless the patient exercises, when the ankle jerks characteristically disappear. This condition may closely mimic intermittent claudication, but the pedal pulses are likely to be palpable. X-rays and ultrasound can be used to assess the width of the canal. If the symptoms are sufficiently distressing, surgical decompression can be undertaken.

Scoliosis

This is a lateral curvature of the spine with rotation of the vertebral bodies. It may be due to a developmental abnormality, or to an acquired disease of the vertebral bodies or muscles. It is important not to miss a developing scoliosis in a young child as intervention can only help before growth has ceased. The best test for a fixed scoliosis is to view the child from the rear as she touches her toes. A postural scoliosis will disappear; a fixed one will show as an asymmetrical rib hump. These children should have early supervision from a spinal unit.

INFLAMMATORY CONDITIONS

Spondylitis, inflammatory joint disease at the spinal joints, is caused by ankylosing spondylitis and others of the B27 antigen associated diseases (see Chapter 4). In its early stages it may closely mimic low back pain of mechanical origin as the following case history illustrates.

Brian T, aged 24, is a self-employed decorator who rarely attends the surgery. He consulted for a bout of low back pain which had interfered with his work. It was worse on lifting and twisting, and he took some time to limber up in the mornings. The pain settled over four weeks, and his next attendance was for a moderate effusion in his left knee which he attributed to football at the weekend. Some months later he had further back pain and some early morning stiffness. His GP thought his lumbar segment was a little rigid and arranged an ESR and sacro-iliac X-ray. These all came back normal. He enrolled in the back life class with the Physiotherapy Department and took up swimming.

Two years later he attended again with a stiff back. Examination showed restricted lateral flexion and pain on stressing the sacro-iliac joints. There were no signs of the other problems associated with ankylosing spondylitis. X-rays showed erosions at the sacro-iliac joint margins and his ESR was 45 mm. He responds well to indomethacin 75 mg at night, and understands the need to exercise regularly and maintain his spinal posture.

OTHER CAUSES OF LOW BACK PAIN

Metabolic disorders

Osteoporosis only causes back pain when microfractures or crush fractures develop. These can occur with minimal trauma and can be extremely painful, taking many weeks to settle.

Osteomalacia may present as low back pain, often with limb pains or generalized aches. It is not uncommon amongst the female Asian population. Screening tests include the alkaline phosphatase which will be elevated, and there is usually a low serum calcium. The diagnosis can be confirmed by finding a low serum vitamin D. The characteristic pseudo-fractures seen on X-rays are best seen on pelvic films. Treatment is with vitamin D (see p. 118).

Paget's disease affecting the spine is usually a chance radiological finding; even a small focus can cause gross elevation of the alkaline phosphatase. Treatment is discussed on page 120.

Tumours and infections

Malignant deposits in the lumbar spine, usually secondaries from breast, prostate, lung, or myelomatosus, are relatively uncommon in general practice but should be considered in the middle-aged or elderly. Pointers to a malignant deposit include:

Local tenderness
Increasing pain unrelieved by rest.

Frequently the symptoms are non-specific in the early weeks or months and X-rays may show no abnormality. If in doubt a bone scan in combination with an ESR and alkaline phosphatase may clarify the situation. Alternatively repeat X-rays a month or two apart may demonstrate changes. Treatment will depend upon the nature of the neoplasm.

Osteomyelitis of the spine is a rare but potentially life-threatening condition. Tuberculosis still remains the commonest cause; other agents include *Staphylococcus, Haemophilus, Salmonella,* and *Brucella* species. Continuous unrelieved pain with restriction of all spinal movements should make one suspicious. There may not always be evidence of systemic upset. Immediate admission should be arranged for intensive antimicrobial therapy.

REFERENCES

Arthritis and Rheumatism Council Handbook for Patients. *Backache* (available from 41 Eagle Street, London WC1R 4AR).
Currey, H. L. F. and Greenwood, R. M. *et al.* (1979). A prospective study of low back pain. *Rheumatol. Rehab.* **18**, 94–104.
Cyriax, J. (1982). *Textbook of orthopaedic medicine.* Vol. 1, 8th edn, Balliere Tindall, London.
Dillane, J. B. and Fry, J. (1966). Acute back syndrome—A study from general practice. *Br. med. J.* **2**, 82–4.
Forrest, A. J. and Wolkind, S. N. (1974). Masked depression in men with low back pain. *Rheum. Rehab.* **13**, 148–53.
Gibson, T., Harkness, J., *et al.* (1985). Controlled comparison of short-wave diathermy treatment with osteophathic treatment in non-specific low back pain. *Lancet* 1258–60.

Roland, M. O., Morrell, D. C., and Morris, R. W. (1983). Can general practitioners predict the outcome of episodes of back pain? *Br. med. J.* **290**, 523–5.

Saad, Z., Nagi, L. E. *et al.* (1973). A social epidemiology of back pain in a general population. *J. Chron. Dis.* **26**, 769–79.

Ward, T., Knowelden, J., and Sharrard, W. J. W. (1968). Low back pain. *J. R. Coll. Gen. Pract.* **15**, 128–36.

12 Regional problems III:

The shoulder

Unlike the hip joint, in which the deep ball-and-socket arrangement produces stability, the shallow gleno-humeral articulation of the shoulder offers little mechanical security. What stability there is comes from the tendons of the scapulohumeral group of muscles which, as they pass across the joint, are expanded into strap-like thickenings of the capsule, the so-called rotator cuff. Additional support comes from the tendon of the long head of the biceps as it passes through the joint cavity, while upward displacement of the humeral head is resisted by the acromion and the coraco-acromial ligament. This arrangement of the glenohumeral joint, combined with the freedom of the scapula to glide and rotate on the chest wall, accounts for the very wide range of circumduction and rotation possible at the shoulder. It may also account for the frequent occurrence of a group of disorders unique to the shoulder and thought to involve the tendons of the scapulohumeral muscles, the rotator cuff, the joint capsule, and related bursae.

Injection of the shoulder

Painful and stiff disorders of the shoulder are common. As explained below, the exact definition of the various clinical conditions remains a matter of debate. Nevertheless, using screening tests such as the ESR it is relatively easy to exclude inflammatory rheumatic, infective, or neoplastic lesions, and the management problem then becomes one of controlling pain and preventing further stiffness. It is in these circumstances that local injections of corticosteroid are tried. These may be dramatically effective in shoulders which are very irritable but have a good range of movement (e.g. supraspinatus or bicipital tendinitis), but are likely to achieve less when there is marked restriction of movement (e.g. frozen shoulder). Nevertheless, patients with painful stiff shoulders deserve at least a trial of injection treatment. Some will require repeated injections. The general practitioner who undertakes these injections in his surgery is able to provide a much more satisfactory service for his patients, not least in avoiding delays and unnecessary visits to hospital. Other points in favour of giving these injections as a surgery procedure are that they are very safe: using standard disposable equipment and a no-touch technique, complications are very rare.

Exact placement of the injected material—while always aimed for—is not necessarily critical: some injections which have clearly not 'hit-the-spot' nevertheless produce a good result, and do no harm.

It is clearly an advantage if the operator can initially obtain some supervised experience, e.g. by attending injection sessions in a hospital rheumatology department. However, this is not essential and the description which follows should enable the general practitioner to undertake shoulder injections on his own.

Technique

The exact target aimed for will depend on the anatomical diagnosis and the site of maximum tenderness. Some examples are mentioned below. However, very often a particular target is not identified and then the injection is given into the region of the sub-acromial bursa. This structure is in close relationship to the capsule and rotator cuff and often communicates with the joint cavity. In the absence of specific indications to inject elsewhere, this is the target to go for (see below for a description of how to inject the joint cavity directly).

The following sequence is designed to give the beginner confidence. Once experience is gained the initial infiltration with local anaesthetic may be omitted in straightforward cases. Alternatively, the lignocaine may be mixed with the corticosteroid in one syringe. Immediate relief of pain on movement then provides a positive check that the injection has reached the source of the pain.

1. Position the patient sitting on a chair with the arm hanging freely down by his side. (In case of faintness the treatment is immediately to get his head down between his knees.)
2. Palpate the shoulder and plan the point of needle entry *before* washing your hands. This is the most important part of the procedure. The bulky deltoid muscle makes the landmarks somewhat difficult to identify at the outermost point of the shoulder (where the needle will enter) therefore start by palpating the acromion posteriorly where the prominent angle is easily felt. (All the shoulder landmarks are easily identified on oneself.) Having located the edge of the acromion, move forwards to the outermost point of the shoulder and feel for the groove between the acromion above and the humerus below. Positive identification is achieved by asking the patient to rotate the arm: the palpating finger should now feel the stationary acromion above and the rotating greater tuberosity of the humerus below. The needle should enter so as to slide between the acromion and the greater tuberosity. Mark this point on the skin.
3. Check that everything necessary is within easy reach. This

includes a sterile, dry swab (in case of bleeding) a small adhesive dressing, and an artery forceps to assist in dislodging needles from syringes.

4. Wash your hands.

5. Draw up 2 ml of lignocaine 1 per cent in a 2 ml syringe. Leave a 23 gauge (blue), 40 mm (1.5 inch) needle in its cover on the syringe.

6. Into a second 2 ml syringe draw up (from a single-dose vial) the corticosteroid preparation to be injected. In the case of hydrocortisone acetate (25 mg/ml) use 50 mg (2 ml). For the various more potent preparations (which some believe to be more effective than hydrocortisone) follow the makers recommendations about dosage. Do not use multi-dose vials for intra-articular injections; they are an infection risk. Leave the needle loosely attached to the syringe.

7. Clean the skin with a swab soaked in an alcohol based antiseptic from a sealed sachet. Allow the skin to dry.

8. A right-handed operator now places the pulps of the index and middle fingers of the left hand (cleaned at the same time as the patient's skin) one in front of and one behind the point of entry of the needle (Fig. 12.1). This confirms the position of the groove between the acromion and humerus. The needle of the syringe containing the local anaesthetic is inserted into the skin, a drop is injected, and the needle is advanced gradually (infiltrating anaesthetic in the process) so that it slides between the acromion and the humerus. If bone or cartilage is struck, the needle is

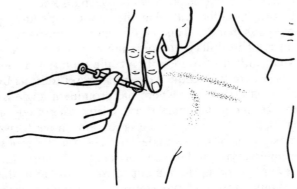

Fig. 12.1. Technique for sub-acromial bursa injection. In the absence of a more specific target this is generally the best site for corticosteroid injections in painful/stiff shoulder conditions. The two fingers of the operator's left hand are locating the groove between the acromion above and the greater tuberosity of the humerus below. The patient should be seated with the arm hanging down freely.

withdrawn slightly and the direction adjusted. Having the area anaesthetic allows this to be done without discomfort to the patient, and the two fingers of the left hand provide general guidance. Advance the needle until it has penetrated to its full length.

9. Remove the syringe from the needle, leaving the latter *in situ*. If the needle is tightly stuck on the syringe use the artery forceps to dislodge it.

10. Take up the syringe containing the corticosteroid and attach it to the needle.

11. 'Draw back' to check that the needle is not in a blood vessel, then inject the contents. Little resistance should be felt on pressing the plunger. Strong resistance may indicate that the needle tip is actually in the supraspinatus tendon, in which case the needle must be moved to another position before injecting.

12. Withdraw the needle. Stop any bleeding by pressure with the gauze swab. Apply a small adhesive dressing.

13. Warn the patient that there may be an initial worsening of pain during the first twelve to twenty-four hours. Light activities with the arm may be undertaken immediately, but heavy activities should be avoided for a week or two, even if the pain has cleared.

The conditions for which this type of injection are employed are generally self-limiting. If a technically satisfactory injection fails to produce improvement, then a repeat injection may be tried two or three weeks later, but is unlikely to be much more successful. If temporary relief is obtained, but pain returns later, then it is worth repeating the injection once or twice, perhaps at three-weekly intervals. Beyond this, further injections are probably not worth trying.

Injecting the shoulder joint directly

When local injection treatment is used for synovitis of the shoulder joint (as in rheumatoid arthritis) the indirect approach through the (communicating) sub-acromial bursa, described above, may be used. Alternatively, the injection may be made directly into the joint cavity via the anterior approach, and this route should be employed when an effusion is to be aspirated. The patient sits with the arm hanging freely down towards the floor and externally rotated. The needle is inserted from the front at a point just below the coracoid process and is slid between the humeral head and the glenoid rim (Fig. 12.2). With careful initial identification of the bony landmarks, this is a relatively straightforward procedure.

A posterior approach to the synovial cavity can also be used.

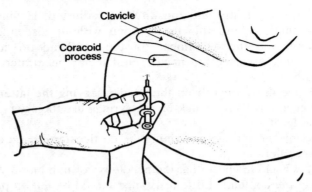

Fig. 12.2. Technique for gleno-humeral joint injection. To enter the shoulder joint directly (e.g. in order to aspirate an effusion), the arm is externally rotated and the needle is inserted anteriorly below the coracoid process.

CAPSULITIS AND FROZEN SHOULDER

As mentioned above, the mechanism and pathology of the extremely common shoulder complaints in which pain and stiffness are the main features, are poorly understood. Certainly the titles used to describe the different clinical patterns imply an exactness of anatomical and patho-logical diagnosis which is seldom justified. The term tendinitis is probably appropriate when tenderness over a tendon or its point of insertion is associated with pain on peforming the movement served by that tendon against resistance. Three examples of tendinitis are discussed below. When the signs are more widespread the terms capsulitis or frozen shoulder are applied. The closely associated sub-acromial bursa is probably involved to some extent in these processes, and some regard 'sub-acromial bursitis' as a separate diagnosis (for a somewhat contro-versial account of these various stiff/painful shoulder conditions treated as separate disorders see Cyriax 1982).

Capsulitis

This term is applied to a common, benign, self-limiting condition of the shoulder in which there is modest limitation of some or all glenohumeral joint movements associated with moderate to severe pain.

Patients are generally middle-aged and describe pain developing in one shoulder (uncommonly both) usually over a period of a few weeks. The symptoms may follow a 'strain' or an episode of trauma, often minor, and the pain is commonly felt in the region of the insertion of the deltoid, rather than the tip of the shoulder. (Pain in the latter site may arise from the acromioclavicular joint or be referred from the diaphragm.) The pain is characteristically worse in bed at night, keeping the patient awake and preventing him sleeping on that side. By day particular manoeuvres produce a sharp stab of pain. Patients learn to put the affected arm into the sleeve of a jacket first and to use the other arm for washing the back.

Examination reveals a shoulder which is neither warm nor swollen (there may be slight wasting of the deltoid). There is likely to be slight to moderate restriction of some or all glenohumeral movements, and these are painful at the limiting positions. Resisted active movement may be particularly uncomfortable. For the assessment of glenohumeral joint movements and for following the progress of these stiff/painful shoulder conditions, the most useful movements to test are passive glenohumeral abduction and internal and external rotation (either with arm by the side or in 90 degrees abduction). X-rays are normal and laboratory tests show no evidence of any systemic disturbance, the ESR, haemoglobin, etc, being unaffected. These tests are employed to exclude conditions (such as myelomatosis or an atypical onset of rheumatoid arthritis) which may mimic shoulder capsulitis.

Perhaps the most characteristic feature of shoulder capsulitis (indeed of all these stiff/painful shoulder conditions) is the fact that it improves spontaneously after a period which averages about eighteen months. In a typical case pain may increasingly dominate the clinical picture during the first six months; the condition then remains static during the second six months, while the final six months are dominated by stiffness without much pain. Eventually there is full resolution of pain, leaving perhaps 10 per cent painless restriction of movement. The nature of the pathology is unknown, but it is assumed to involve the capsule and related structures, rather than the synovium.

Management is often less than satisfactory. Some relief of pain may be obtained by analgesics and electric hot pads, and it is worth trying the effect of one or more injections of local corticosteroid into the region of the sub-acromial bursa (see p. 154). The degree of relief obtained ranges from negligible to moderate. Physiotherapy in a variety of forms is traditionally tried, but benefit has never been proven. In particularly troublesome cases, low-dose X-ray therapy may be tried but, again, the value is unproven. As far as physical activity goes the traditional advice is to 'keep the shoulder moving' within the pain-free range, but to avoid manoeuvres which provoke pain. Manipulation under anaesthesia is sometimes undertaken. Its value is unproven and there is a suspicion that it may worsen an irritable shoulder. One rather aggressive form of treatment which has not been adequately tested is the administration of systemic corticosteroids (with or without manipulation) early in the course of severe capsulitis.

Frozen shoulder (adhesive capsulitis)

It is uncertain whether frozen shoulder is a different disorder from capsulitis, or a more severe form of the same condition. It differs from capsulitis in that it affects older patients, glenohumeral movements are almost completely abolished, pain is more severe, and the condition is more often precipitated by some other medical or surgical event.

Some of the preciptating factors have in common the fact that they cause pain and/or immobility of the arm. Examples are herpes zoster, a stroke, or a mastectomy. Other cases appear to be precipitated by more or less silent intrathoracic events such as carcinoma of the lung or myocardial ischaemia.

The pain may become intolerably severe and these elderly patients may become suicidally depressed. As with capsulitis, the pain is worse at night and it may be impossible to sleep on the affected side. It differs from capsulitis in that, on examination, the glenohumeral joint is almost completely fixed: attempts to move it produce a sensation approaching that of fibrous ankylosis. If the strict diagnostic criteria of extreme fixation is applied, then frozen shoulder is much less common than capsulitis.

The natural history of frozen shoulder is similar to that of capsulitis. The condition is self-limiting, and settles eventually after an average duration of about eighteeen months to leave a slightly stiff—but painless—joint.

Treatment is along similar lines to that for capsulitis, except that there is a strong suspicion that prevention may be possible. On the assumption that immobility is often an important aetiological factor, patients who have recently experienced a stroke, zoster affecting an arm, or a mastectomy, are treated by early mobilization of the shoulder on that side, using both passive and (when possible) active arm exercises. In the established case, unfortunately, most of the measures mentioned for capsulitis are likely to be tried in sequence until eventually the condition runs its natural course and the pain settles. Recurrences on the same side are uncommon, but the two sides are occasionally involved in sequence.

The shoulder–hand syndrome

This represents a rare extension, or complication, of the clinical picture of frozen shoulder. In this the frozen shoulder is accompanied by painful swelling, stiffness, and an actual small joint arthropathy affecting the hand on that side. The pain is distressingly intractable and 'causalgic' in character, and the hand is held protectively against the waist, immobile, with the fingers partly flexed. The skin of the hand shows evidence of autonomic changes, with moist, cold skin and cyanosis. This probably represents a more severe ('fuller expression') of the frozen shoulder syndrome. Treatment is similar, except that a cervical sympathetic block is sometimes tried. Eventual resolution can be expected, but this may take months or years and leave some residual shoulder and hand stiffness.

TENDINITIS

As mentioned above, amongst the various stiff/painful shoulder conditions, the term tendinitis is used when pain is provoked by the patient performing—against resistance—the particular movement served by the tendon in question. There may also be tenderness over the tendon, or its point of insertion, while passive shoulder movements are generally well retained. Three common forms of tendinitis are recognized (Table 12.1 and Fig. 12.3).

1. *Supraspinatus tendinitis* is much the most common. Maximal tenderness is over the tip of the greater tuberosity, resisted abduction provokes the pain, and most patients exhibit the sign of the 'painful arc' (Fig. 12.4): on active total abduction of the arm pain is experienced between the 60 degree and 120 degree positions. Relief of pain on passing the 120 degree position corresponds with the moment when the patient rotates the arm externally into the palm-up position. This confirms that one element in production of this pain is impingement of the greater tuberosity against the structures above: the acromion and/or coraco-acromial ligament. The condition has to be differentiated from rupture of the supraspinatus tendon in which initiation of

Table 12.1. *Three common forms of tendinitis of the shoulder (see also Fig. 12.3)*

	Painful active (resisted) movement	Point of maximum tenderness	Other features
Supraspinatus tendinitis	Abduction	Tip of greater tuberosity	'Painful arc' (Fig. 12.4) Occasionally radiological calcification round tendon
Bicipital tendinitis	Elbow flexion Forearm supination	Bicipital groove	
Infraspinatus tendinitis	External rotation	Greater tuberosity (behind and below the tip)	

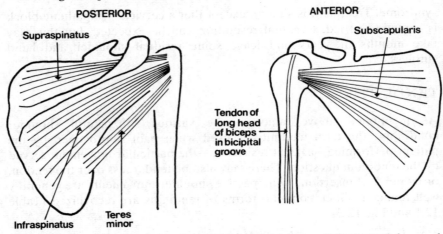

Fig. 12.3. Diagrammatic anterior and posterior views of the scapulohumeral muscles most commonly involved in tendinitis lesions.

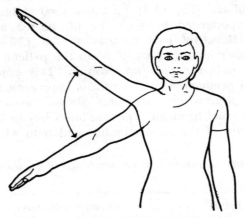

Fig. 12.4. The 'painful arc' of supraspinatus tendinitis. The arrow indicates the range of active abduction through which pain is felt.

active abduction of the shoulder is lost. (An intact deltoid can complete abduction after the first 20 degrees.)

In straightforward cases of supraspinatus tendinitis X-rays are usually normal, but occasionally they show a highly characteristic deposit of calcific material around the distal part of the supraspinatus tendon (above or medial to the greater tuberosity). Shoulders showing this radiological sign may experience extremely acute and severe pain. During the course of an attack ('acute calcific supraspinatus tendinitis') serial X-rays over a few days may show the fragmentation and sometimes complete disappearance of the calcific deposit, pointing to the likelihood that such acute attacks represent an inflammatory reaction to released crytals of hydroxy-apatite. (Very rarely similar attacks may effect various joints at different times: 'multiple calcific peri-arthritis'.)

Supraspinatus tendinitis is more responsive to treatment than other painful/stiff shoulder conditions. An injection of 2 ml hydro-cortisone (25 mg/ml) into the region of the supraspinatus tendon (but not into the body of the tendon itself) can be dramatically effective. The hydrocortisone should be deposited around the site of maximal tenderness, or into the site of radiological calcification or—if neither of these pointers is present—insert the needle as for sub-acromial bursa injection (p. 154) and inject the contents of the syringe along the full length of the needle track as it is withdrawn. Symptomatic treatment may be needed in addition, as described above for capsulitis.

2. *Bicipital tendinitis* is less common. Pain down the front of the upper arm is aggravated by resisted flexion of the elbow or supination of the forearm with the elbow flexed to 90 degrees. Passive movements are usually reasonably well maintained. Tenderness is maximal over the tendon as it lies in the bicipital groove in front of the upper humerus (Fig. 12.3).

This groove can usually be identified by deep palpation in the anterior aspect of the upper humerus while the arm is rotated alternately in and out. Bicipital tendinitis has to be differentiated from rupture of the long head of biceps which may present a somewhat similar picture but, in addition, flexion of the elbow against resistance causes a striking 'ball' of tense muscle to bulge out of the belly of the biceps muscle.

Treatment is generally satisfactory. Two millilitres of hydro-cortisone (25 mg/ml) should be injected into the site of maximum tenderness in the bicipital groove. The injection may have to be repeated, and symptomatic treatment for the relief of pain may also be needed.

3. *Infraspinatus tendinitis* (Table 12.1 and Fig. 12.3) is somewhat similar to bicipital tendinitis, but the diagnosis is generally less clear-cut. Characteristically tenderness should be maximal over a point on the greater tuberosity just behind and below the tip and pain should be provoked by active external rotation against resistance. Treatment is similar to the other types of tendinitis, the injection of corticosteroid being directed to the maximal site of tenderness behind and below the tip of the greater tuberosity.

Table 12.2. *Some pointers in the differential diagnosis of stiff/painful shoulder conditions*

Painful stiff shoulder conditions	**ESR elevated**	Marked early morning stiffness (usually bilateral)	Latex positive → Definite joint limitation →	Rheumatoid arthritis
			Latex negative →	Seronegative polyarthritis
		Unimpressive early morning stiffness	No true limitation →	Polymyalgia rheumatica
				Tuberculosis and other infections
				Myelomatosis
				Secondary deposits
	ESR normal (usually unilateral)	Marked pain and restriction in all directions →		Frozen Shoulder
		Modest pain and restriction in all directions →		Capsulitis
		Relatively full movement but pain on executing one movement against resistance. Tender over tendon involved →		Tendinitis (various)
		Progressive destructive arthritis with recurrent effusions (often haemorrhagic sometimes containing crystals) →		Degenerative shoulder arthritis in elderly

The major diagnostic problem is usually to decide whether pain arises in the shoulder or whether it is referred from the cervical spine. As a general rule all the conditions discussed in this chapter are associated with either some restriction of shoulder joint movement or with pain on movement (full passive movements and resisted active movements). If careful examination reveals neither of these physical signs then the pain probably arises elsewhere.

As with all skeletal pains, it is important to remember that both secondary carcinomatous deposits and metabolic bone disease (p. 114) are uncommon but important mimics of rheumatic conditions. X-rays of the shoulders rarely contribute to the diagnosis (unless there is a specific pointer to the need for this investigation). By contrast a chest X-ray is a useful screening test

DEGENERATIVE SHOULDER CONDITIONS

The shoulder joint, so commonly involved in rheumatoid arthritis, is uncommonly affected by primary osteoarthritis. However, trauma may lead to secondary osteoarthritis. In addition, one occasionally encounters rather destructive and disabling shoulder lesions in the elderly which appear to be 'primary' and mainly degenerative. Typically such patients present with increasing pain and restriction of—usually—one shoulder, with an obvious effusion. Aspiration reveals a synovial fluid which is often blood-stained, and in which various crystals—including pyrophosphate and/or hydroxyapatite—may be identified. X-rays show a destructive type of degenerative change, and sometimes calcification of the capsule or other structures. The mechanism of this unusual type of arthropathy in the elderly is not understood. Whether 'crystal synovitis' is the primary event, or whether trauma or wear and tear lead to crystal deposition is unknown. Variations of this clinical picture have been described as 'l'epaule senile hemorrhagique' and 'Milwaukee shoulder'. For a recent review of the topic see Dieppe *et al.*, 1984.

Treatment is unsatisfactory. Following aspiration effusions tend to re-accumulate, and joint damage is liable to progress to a destructive arthropathy with chronic pain and persistent effusion.

Table 12.2 gives some pointers to the differential diagnosis of stiff/painful shoulders.

ACROMIOCLAVICULAR JOINT LESIONS

When a patient points to the tip of the shoulder as the site of pain, this often indicates that the pain originates, not in the glenohumeral articulation, but from either the acromioclavicular joint or the diaphragm. Diaphragmatic pain is usually clearly related to respiration. Lesions of the acromioclavicular joint are identified by local tenderness and pain on movement (shrugging the shoulders moves both the acromioclavicular and the sternoclavicular joints). The commonest lesions are strains or traumatic subluxations. If pain persists despite rest, a local corticosteroid injection may be tried. Occasionally these joints may be involved in arthropathies such as ankylosing spondylitis.

REFERENCES

Apley, A. G. and Solomon, L. (1982). *Apley's System of Orthopaedics and Fractures.* (6th edn). Butterworths, London.

Cyriax, J. (1982). *Textbook of Orthopaedic Medicine.* Vol. 1. (8th edn). Balliere Tindall, London.

Dieppe, P. A., Doherty, M., Macfarlane, D. G., Hutton, C. W., *et al.*, (1984). Apatite associated destructive arthritis. *Br. J. Rheumatol.* **23**, 84–91.

13 Regional problems IV:

The upper limb

Common rheumatological problems in the arm and hand derive either from local pathology or from disease in the neck, shoulder or lungs. Hence, although local examination is quite adequate for many conditions, it is important to look for more distant pathology if the cause of the problem is not immediately obvious. For example, cervical spondylosis may cause root pain in the arm with little neck pain; a Pancoast's tumour in the apex of the lung may cause root pain or weakness in the arm by eroding the lower branches of the brachial plexus; and a patient with a frozen shoulder will occasionally complain of pain in the upper arm.

Functional anatomy

The humero-ulnar joint at the elbow is a simple hinge, allowing flexion and extension only. Rotation of the forearm is achieved at the proximal radiohumeral and the distal radio-ulnar joints. When examining the range of movement in the elbow, wrist and hands, comparison with the other limb is the most useful guide to the expected range since there is considerable variation in joint mobility between individuals, and a natural decline with age. The most complex knowledge required of the upper limb relates to the distribution of dermatomes and the muscles supplied by the three principal peripheral nerves. The details are difficult to remember if they are not used daily, so a dermatome chart (Fig. 10.2) to hang in the surgery, along with a chart of peripheral nerves and the muscles they supply, is useful. (Table 10.3, p. 128.)

The radial nerve

The radial nerve ($C_{5,6,7}$) is most commonly damaged by mid-shaft fractures of the humerus, or by pressure in the axilla on the lowest roots of the brachial plexus (crutch paralysis). The motor component of this nerve supplies the extensor muscles of the hand. Simple quick tests for motor function include resisted extension of the wrist and extension of the thumb (Fig. 13.1). The sensory distribution covers a small area on the back of the hand between the thumb and index finger.

The median nerve

The median nerve ($C_{6,7,8}$ T_1) may be damaged as it passes through the carpal tunnel to enter the hand. It can also be damaged by prolonged

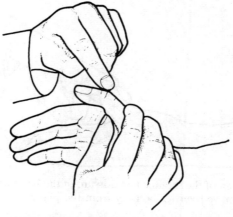

Fig. 13.1. Testing extension of the thumb. It is important to test extension at the carpometacarpal joint, since interphalangeal extension can be achieved by the intrinsic muscles.

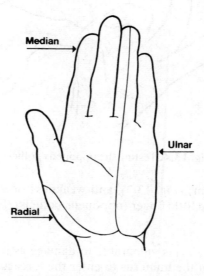

Fig. 13.2. The sensory distribution of the three nerves to the hand.

pressure in the palm. Its motor component supplies most of the flexor aspect of the forearm, and the muscles of the thenar eminence. Trauma to the nerve above the wrist will cause weakness of wrist and finger flexion. The common lesion in medical neurology is the carpal tunnel syndrome. Pressure on the nerve at this level causes weakness of abductor pollicis brevis (weakness on abduction of the thumb away from

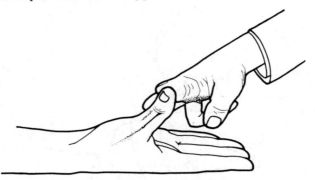

Fig. 13.3. Abduction of the thumb. The dorsum of the hand lies on a flat surface, and the thumb is moved vertically away from the plane of the palm to test this movement.

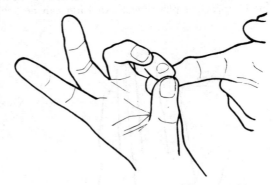

Fig. 13.4. Testing the opponens pollicis.

the plane of the palm) (Fig. 13.3), and weakness on attempting opposition of the thumb and little finger (opponens pollicis) (Fig. 13.4).

The ulnar nerve

The ulnar nerve (C_8, T_1) is vulnerable to damage as it passes behind the medial epicondyle of the humerus to enter the forearm. Its motor supply is to the majority of the intrinsic muscles of the hand. Paralysis of the nerve causes the characteristic claw hand, in which the ring and little finger are semi-flexed by the action of the flexor digitorum muscle which is unopposed due to loss of the interossei and lumbrical action. The most reliable test of ulnar nerve function is abduction of the little finger. Abduction and adduction of the other digits is also affected, but in certain positions of the fingers the long flexors and extensors can achieve these movements, so this test should be performed with the palm on a flat surface.

If the distribution of weakness or sensory loss does not fit one of these patterns, consider a cervical root lesion (p. 127), or a peripheral neuropathy.

TENDONS AND LIGAMENTS

Tennis elbow (lateral humeral epicondylitis)

This condition is one of several in which there is a painful inflammatory reaction at the junction of tendon and bone. In this case the painful site is at the junction of the fibrous portion of the common extensor origin with the lateral humeral epicondyle. The cause is obscure, and an obvious precipitating event rarely precedes it, although in some cases there may be small tears in the fibrous extensor origin. It affects adults of all ages but there is peak incidence between the ages of 40 and 60.

If the condition is mild the patient describes an ache around the elbow brought on by certain twisting or lifting movements. In severe cases the pain distribution widens, spreading towards the wrist and shoulder, and there may be a constant dull ache. Examination shows a normal range of movement at the elbow joint, but a painful spot on palpation over the lateral humeral epicondyle. Resisted dorsiflexion of the wrist will bring on the pain. With no treatment the condition tends to wax and wane over several months and eventually clear up. The occasional severe case will cause persistent pain and loss of function over months or even years.

Initial treatment consists of a local steroid injection. Hydrocortisone acetate is recommended rather than the stronger or longer-acting steroid preparations which may cause atrophy of the overlying skin. The needle is inserted at the point of maximum tenderness, into the fibrous origin of the extensor muscles overlying the lateral epicondyle (Fig. 13.5). Some authorities consider that multiple small deposits of steroid at different

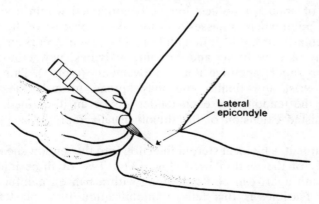

Fig. 13.5. Injection site for tennis elbow.

sites under the skin have more chance of effecting a cure first time. This is a very safe procedure; so long as the hands are washed and the skin cleaned with an antiseptic, little damage can be done. Apart from inserting the needle into bone (when injection will be impossible) there are no immediate adjacent structures which can be damaged.

The patient should be warned that the pain may be worse for the first few days, and advised to avoid painful movements if this is possible. Over a period of two weeks it will become clear whether or not the injection has helped. About 50 per cent improve after a first injection. It is the authors' practice to give up to three or four injections at about monthly intervals. If the condition remains painful after that time the following options may be tried:

Await natural resolution.
Firm strapping below the elbow, or splinting.
Trial of physiotherapy; ultrasound is occasionally helpful.
Consider surgical referral. This may be necessary in obstinate cases.

Golfer's elbow: Medial humeral epicondylitis

This is an exactly analogous, although much less common, condition affecting the common flexor origin on the medial epicondyle. Resisted wrist flexion will reproduce the pain, and a tender spot can be palpated over the medial epicondyle. Treatment is similar to that for tennis elbow, but when planning the point of injection one should keep away from the ulnar nerve which runs in the groove behind the medial humeral epicondyle.

De Quervain's syndrome: tenosynovitis of abductor pollicis longus

The tendon of abductor pollicis longus is contained within a synovial tunnel at the point where it passes over the styloid process of the radius, and is particularly prone to inflammation. This often occurs in people who suddenly take on lifting and wringing activities (new mothers) or those who do rapid repetitive thumb movements (typists). Pain is felt around the wrist and thumb and may spread towards the elbow. Palpation of the tendon may elicit tenderness or an ill-defined, boggy swelling. Resisted extension of the thumb usually reproduces the pain (Fig. 13.1).

Initial treatment is by local steroid injection into the tendon sheath, not into the body of the tendon itself (Fig. 13.6). Two or three injections spaced a month apart can be tried, along with a ban on painful movements when feasible. If this fails, immobilization in a plaster cast, extending from the mid-forearm to the distal skin crease of the thumb,

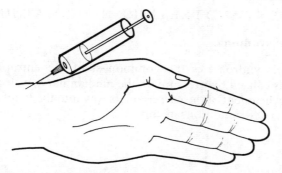

Fig. 13.6. Injection site for de Quervain's tenosynovitis.

for six weeks may allow the inflammation to subside. If this too is unsuccessful, surgical incision of the tendon sheath is usually curative.

Trigger finger: (stenosing tenovaginitis)

Trigger finger is a thickening of one of the flexor tendons of the fingers. The commonest association is with rheumatoid arthritis. The patient complains that the finger 'sticks' in partial flexion. A sharp pull will overcome the obstruction and it will snap open or shut. Palpation of the palm as the patient performs this manoeuvre usually shows that the thickening lies over one of the metacarpal heads. Treatment is by one or two local steroid injections into the tendon sheath at the site of the thickening. If this fails surgical release is curative.

BURSAE

Olecranon bursitis

The bursa overlying the olecranon process readily becomes inflamed. This inflammation may be associated with rheumatoid arthritis, when nodules may be felt within the swelling. A simple bursitis can take months to settle naturally. Aspiration (if the contents are not too viscous) and injection with a steroid preparation may halt the inflammatory process. If not, and the bursa is sufficiently troublesome, surgical removal is occasionally needed.

An inflamed bursa may be infected or gouty. Fluid can be removed for culture and crystal examination; antibiotics should be started while the results are awaited. Rheumatoid bursitis rarely settles if the disease is in an active phase.

ENTRAPMENT AND PRESSURE NEUROPATHIES

Carpal tunnel syndrome

Carpal tunnel syndrome is the commonest of the entrapment neuro-pathies, and is caused by pressure on the median nerve as it passes under the transverse ligament of the carpus on its way into the hand (Fig. 13.7). Some associated conditions include:

Obesity
Pregnancy
Myxoedema
Rheumatoid arthritis
Acromegaly

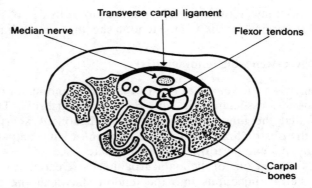

Fig. 13.7. Cross section of the wrist to show the structures surrounding the median nerve.

The history is usually characteristic. The patient reports numbness or an aching sensation in the hand with tingling in the fingers. Sometimes the aching pain spreads up the forearm to the elbow. It often wakes the patient at night, but in this instance relief may be obtained by hanging the arm out of bed and wringing the hand. The numb sensation may be described by the patient as clumsiness or weakness, but objective evidence of weakness in uncommon. Sensory impairment in the distribu-tion of the median nerve should be sought, as should loss of muscle bulk in the thenar eminence. Tests for abductor pollicis brevis (Fig. 13.3) and opponens pollicis (Fig. 13.4), both supplied by the median nerve, will demonstrate any weakness if it is present. Tinel's sign (tapping over the middle of the wrist to produce tingling in the median nerve distribution) is not often positive in mild cases. If the history is clearcut, treatment should begin before there is evidence of weakness or wasting. Mild cases usually respond to either of the following:

1. A wrist splint worn at night to hold the wrist in the neutral or slightly extended position.
2. One or two injections of a soluble steroid preparation into the carpal tunnel.

The site of the injection is at the distal carpal crease (Fig. 13.8), just to the radial side of the palmaris tendon (if present). A volume of soluble steroid preparation not greater than 1 ml should be given. Do not inject if insertion of the needle causes paraesthesia; the point of the needle may be in the nerve. If a fine needle is used, local anaesthetic is rarely necessary. The needle is inserted at an angle of 45 degrees to the skin surface, to a depth of about 0.5–1 cm when it should lie within the carpal tunnel. The patient commonly reports tingling as the injection goes in. This occurs as the fluid fills the space and compresses the nerve. Symptoms may be worse for one or two days after an injection, and any useful effects will be apparent within two weeks.

The patient should be referred for surgical release of the transverse ligament if:

(a) There are objective signs of weakness or wasting.
(b) Electromyography reveals a prolonged latency of conduction between the wrist and abductor pollicis brevis. There may also be electrical evidence of partial denervation.
(c) Two local injections and the use of night splints fail to control the symptoms.

The ulnar nerve

The ulnar nerve lies in a vulnerable position beneath the skin as it runs in the groove on the posterior surface of the medial epicondyle. Distortion of the elbow joint either by trauma or by rheumatoid or osteoarthritis may cause pressure on the nerve at this site, or may stimulate the development of fibrous adhesions around the nerve. This may cause

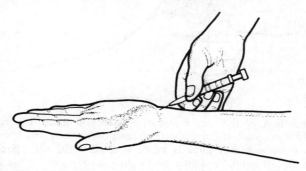

Fig. 13.8. Injection site for carpal tunnel syndrome.

paraesthesia in the ulnar sensory distribution, and if the condition is progressive an ulnar palsy gradually develops, with the characteristic claw hand (see p. 168). Electromyography may be useful in the early stages since the symptoms are often poorly localized. If the symptoms are mild, it may be adequate to persuade the patient to stop leaning on his elbows and to change other habits which cause pressure on the nerve. If not, surgical transposition may be necessary.

ARTHRITIS

Any of the inflammatory arthropathies can affect the joints of the forearm and hand. Stiffness and synovitis of the small joints of the fingers and wrist are a common presenting feature of rheumatoid arthritis, SLE, and the seronegative arthritides. Details of examination and the commoner hand deformities are to be found in the chapters dealing with these conditions.

Two manifestations of osteoarthitis deserve special mention here:

Osteoarthritis of the first carpometacarpal joint

This is a common manifestation of osteoarthritis, forming part of the familial pattern of osteoarthritis in women which includes Heberden's nodes. It may be the only joint of which the patient complains. Pain at the base of the thumb is brought on by repetitive movements of the thumb or normal domestic work. Examination will produce pain on putting the joint through its range of movement. If more severe there may be local

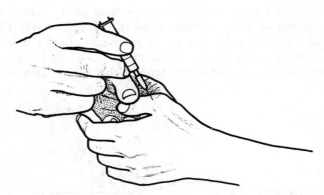

Fig. 13.9. Injection of the first metacarpophalangeal joint. The technique is straightfoward if the joint can be opened by traction on the distal bone. Here the thumb metacarpophalangeal joint is being entered while the operator exerts traction with his left hand. A similar technique can be used for the first carpo-metacarpal joint and the interphalangeal joints.

swelling, crepitus, and subluxation of the joint to produce the 'square-hand' deformity (Fig. 2.8). Usually the pain comes and goes in cycles of weeks or months, and can be controlled with non-steroidal anti-inflammatory drugs. If pain becomes persistent a light splint can be made in the occupational therapy department. This will fixate the painful joint but allow enough use of the thumb for everyday activities. An occasional severe exacerbation of pain may be helped by an intra-articular steroid injection.

Heberden's nodes

Usually these osteophytes on the distal phalanges of the fingers develop insidiously and painlessly, but on occasion a fusiform synovitis predates their arrival. Heberden's nodes may become inflamed, usually during a flare up of the 'inflammatory phase' of osteoarthritis. The inflammation settles with the use of non-steroidal anti-inflammatory drugs or, if persistent, a local steroid injection.

REFERENCES

Boyle, A. C. Local injection of steroids. In *Reports on rheumatic diseases: Collected reports 1959–1983*. Arthritis and Rheumatism Council, London.

14 Regional problems V:
The hip and knee

THE HIP

Anatomy

The deep ball-and-socket arrangement of the hip joint (with the socket further deepened by the labrum acetabulare) provides greater stability, at the cost of reduced mobility, compared with the shoulder. The surface marking of the joint is directly under the mid-point of the inguinal ligament. However, it is important to remember that pain arising in the hip may be felt as referred pain in the knee due to both joints receiving articular branches from the obturator nerve. Occasionally hip joint pathology may produce pain exclusively in the knee, easily leading to serious diagnostic errors.

An important aspect of the anatomy of the hip is the fact that the head of the femur obtains its blood supply almost exclusively from arteries running up the neck of the bone. Anything which interferes with this blood supply is liable to produce ischaemic necrosis of part or all of the head.

Examination of the hip

Inspect the patient—stripped to underclothing—both standing and walking. Differences in leg length may be detected, usually due to pathology in or about the hip. Confirm any difference with the patient lying supine, and with the two legs at the same angle in relationship to the pelvis. Use a tape measure to record the distance between the anterior superior iliac spine and the medial malleolus (Fig. 14.1). A useful screening test for significant hip joint pathology is the *Trendelenberg test* (Fig. 14.2). This depends on the fact that the normal redistribution of weight when lifting one foot off the ground is disturbed when either the hip joint is irritable or unstable, or the muscles acting across the joint are weak. A positive test is usually associated with a 'Trendelenburg gait', in which the opposite side of the pelvis sags during each step while the affected leg is weight-bearing. It is unusual for hip joint effusions to be detected clinically.

Next get the patient onto the couch. For adequate examination of the

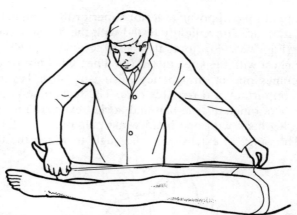

Fig. 14.1. Measuring leg length. The measurement is taken from the anterior superior iliac spine to the medial malleolus. It is critical that the measurements be made with the two legs in the same position in relationship to the pelvis.

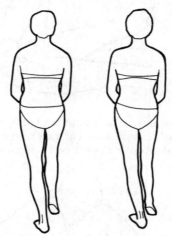

Fig. 14.2. Trendelberg test. On the left is the normal pelvic tilt adopted when standing on one leg. On the right is the sagging of the pelvis on the non-weight-bearing side which represents a positive test result. A positive test may indicate disease of the hip joint or weakness of the muscles on the weight-bearing side.

hip joint the couch must be well clear of the wall on both sides, and an assistant will be required if the patient is disabled or obese.

For testing the range of hip movements it is necessary to bear in mind that, as at the shoulder, true ball-and-socket movement has to be differentiated from movement of the pelvic girdle. Pelvic movement can be detected by observing the position of the anterior superior iliac spines. Thus, in testing the range of adduction and abduction (Fig. 14.3), the examiner palpates the opposite anterior superior iliac spine. Internal and external rotation are conveniently tested with the hip and knee flexed to 90 degrees (Fig. 2.3). Hip joint flexion is tested by pushing the thigh towards the chest with the knee flexed (the knee must not be extended or the test becomes one of straight leg raising p. 140). Testing hip joint extension is important and requires care. The technique is illustrated in Figure 14.4. The range of true ball-and-socket extension is estimated by drawing the leg back with one hand while palpating the iliac crest with the other. The range of extension is the angle to which the thigh can be

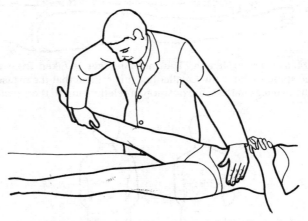

Fig. 14.3. Testing hip abduction. The examiner's left hand on the opposite iliac crest monitors the position of the pelvis. The range of abduction is the angle to which the leg can be carried before the pelvis begins to move with the leg.

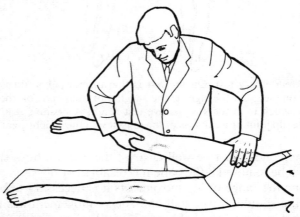

Fig. 14.4. Testing hip extension. The left hand monitors the position of the pelvis. The range of extension is the angle to which the leg can be carried back before the pelvis begins to move with the leg.

drawn back before further movement is achieved by rotation of the pelvis.

A popular manoeuvre in examining the hip is known as Thomas's test. It is illustrated in Figure 14.5. It is particularly valuable in children with hip joint pathology since a mobile lumbar spine may allow a flexion deformity to be 'concealed' by rotation of the pelvis. Abolishing this lumbar lordosis by forcing the opposite thigh up onto the chest reveals the flexion deformity. Abolition of the lumbar lordosis is confirmed by the left hand held in the small of the back. As the lumbar lordosis is abolished, the knee on the affected side rises off the couch to reveal the flexion deformity.

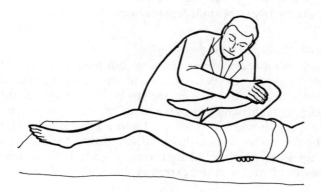

Fig. 14.5. Thomas' test. This test is used to reveal a flexion deformity of the hip joint when the hip flexion is concealed by compensatory lordosis of the lumbar spine. By forced flexion of the *opposite* hip the examiner abolishes the lumbar lordosis (confirmed by a hand in the small of the back) and this causes the flexion deformity to be revealed.

A position of flexion is adopted by the inflamed hip because, in that position, the intra-capsular volume is maximal and hence the joint is under minimum tension. It is important to remember that an apparent flexion deformity of the hip may really be due to psoas muscle spasm resulting from intra-abdominal or lumbar spine pathology (e.g. tuberculosis).

The pattern of hip joint deformity following trauma may occasionally give an initial pointer to the diagnosis: both dislocation of the hip and fracture of the neck of femur produce an apparent shortening of the leg. In the case of a fractured neck of femur the leg rolls outwards so that the lateral border of the foot lies along the ground; with dislocation the hip is partially flexed and internally rotated so that the sole of the affected foot comes to lie upon the dorsum of the opposite foot.

Causes of pain in the hip

Laymen are often uncertain of the anatomical site of the hip, and it is advisable to get the patient to point to the actual distribution of the pain. Hip joint pathology generally produces pain in the groin and down the inner aspect of the thigh. However, as mentioned above, it may also be felt (sometimes exclusively) as pain in the knee. Patients will often ascribe pain in the buttock to hip problems when in fact it arises in the lumbar spine. Table 14.1 lists some of the more important and common causes of 'hip' pain.

Most of these conditions are covered systematically in other chapters of this book. A few points on each disorder are mentioned here to highlight particularly important regional aspects.

Osteoarthritis of the hip (see also Chapter 2)

This is much the most common cause of hip pain in adults. The pain is usually felt in the groin, occasionally in the knee, on the same side. Initially pains occur only during weight-bearing. Later there is spontaneous pain at night which progresses to the point where it interferes with sleep. Usually one hip is affected and joints elsewhere are normal unless it be for nodal osteoarthritis in the hands (p. 21). Examination reveals a hip joint which is, at first, only slightly limited in movement, being somewhat irritable at the extremes. Later these signs become more

Table 14.1. *Some important causes of hip joint pain and some conditions which can mimic hip joint symptoms*

Generally gradual in onset	Osteoarthritis Rheumatoid arthritis Seronegative arthritis (e.g. ankylosing spondylitis) Tuberculosis
May be dramatically acute in onset	Aseptic necrosis Septic arthritis Crystal arthritis Acute flares of inflammatory arthritis Loose fragment
Conditions which may mimic pain arising in the hip joint	Referred root pains Psoas irritation Fracture of neck of femur Bursitis (e.g. trochanteric) Tendinitis Malignant bone deposits Metabolic bone disease

gross, and some loss of leg length points to destructive bony changes. The diagnosis is readily made: the ESR is normal, and the X-ray changes (usually apparent by the time the patient presents) are characteristic (p. 15). The extent of articular cartilage loss is the most useful radiological index of the extent of joint damage. A single conventional film of the pelvis is usually adequate.

Because the early stages of osteoarthritis are painless (articular cartilage being insensitive), the pathological process is usually well advanced by the time the patient first presents. Progress from then onwards is variable. Some patients can be 'kept going' with the use of non-steroidal anti-inflammatory drugs and analgesics. Once a limp develops a walking stick (held in the *opposite* hand) may be helpful (a cane of the correct length should reach the top of the greater trochanter on the normal side). Some patients benefit from instruction in walking with a stick from a physiotherapist, and if 2 cm or more of leg length is lost it is worth trying the effect of a heel raise. Regular prone lying (20 minutes each night) will help to prevent the development of a flexion deformity. Other forms of physiotherapy are not of proven value, although exercises and hydrotherapy are often prescribed.

Total (prosthetic) hip replacement provides the answer for patients aged 60 or over who progress to the point where pain and disability become unacceptable. Once night pain keeps the patient awake this should be considered. However, the limited life of the presently available prostheses makes total hip replacement increasingly less attractive the younger a patient is. Secondary osteoarthritis in a young adult can be treated by arthrodesis (although this may interfere with sexual activity in females), and osteotomy sometimes 'buys time' in a younger patient with primary osteoarthritis of the hip.

Rhematoid arthritis of the hip (see also Chapter 3)

The hip is fortunately not one of the most commonly affected joints in rheumatoid arthritis; however, when it does become involved the disease may progress to produce very severe incapacity. A single hip can be effectively treated by prosthetic replacement (arthrodesis is avoided because of the risk of the opposite hip and knees becoming involved). When both hips and knees are involved in the same patient the situation is much more difficult. Starting a programme of surgery which may finish with the replacement of all four joints is almost too daunting to contemplate.

Seronegative spondarthritis involving the hip (see also Chapter 4)

In an adult with ankylosing spondylitis, involvement of the hip joint carries a bad prognosis. It is likely to prove more troublesome than the spine and is unlikely to respond so well to anti-inflammatory drugs and exercises. Furthermore, unlike the spine, the affected peripheral joint is unresponsive to X-ray treatment. Finally, total hip replacement is likely to be unsatisfactory, not only because the patient is too young for the procedure (see above under osteoarthritis) but also because the general tendency to periosteal new bone overgrowth tends to affect the operation site and interfere with hip movement.

Tuberculosis (see also Chapter 8)

Tuberculous infection of the hip needs to be considered, especially in patients of Asian extraction. Night sweats may provide a clue, but the safe rule is always to carry out an ESR in anyone suffering from skeletal pains. If X-rays and other evidence point to the possibility of tuberculosis it may be necessary to perform a synovial biopsy to obtain material for histology and culture (including drug-sensitivity testing).

Aseptic necrosis of the hip

Attention has been drawn (p. 176) to the somewhat precarious provision of blood to the head of the femur. Interference with this may lead to necrosis of part or all of the femoral head.

The disorder may arise without apparent cause; more often it appears in association with one of the following:

Corticosteroid therapy.	Renal transplantation.
Haemoglobinopathy.	Alcoholism.
Rheumatoid arthritis.	Caisson (decompression) disease.
Fractured neck of femur.	Systemic lupus erythematosus.
Pancreatic disease.	

The pain may be dramatically acute, coming on as the body weight is loaded onto the affected side. Early X-rays may show no change. Later there is evidence of a shallow wedge of subcortical bone separating and collapsing. The upper pole of the joint space is generally well retained. Later there is remodelling of the head, with secondary osteoarthritis. The earliest evidence of aseptic necrosis may be obtained from a radioisotope scan. The avascular area is 'cold' while the interface between the live and dead bone is 'hot'. The lesions vary greatly in size. The larger ones produce severe pain and gross disability. Treatment involves avoiding weight-bearing for a few weeks. Mild cases can resolve to leave a usable hip; severe cases may require prosthetic replacement. Other joints (e.g. shoulder or elbow) may occasionally be involved.

Septic arthritis (see also Chapter 8)

Pyogenic arthritis of the hip is most common in children and represents a medical emergency. It must be suspected in any acute monarthritis of the joint. Early X-rays are generally unhelpful. Immediate transfer to hospital is required and it is essential to delay giving antimicrobial treatment until both blood and synovial fluid have been obtained for microbiological studies.

Crystal arthritis (see also Chapter 5)

For practical purposes gout never involves the hip joint, but pseudo-gout (pyrophosphate arthropathy) may do so. A useful screening test is to X-ray the knees for evidence of chondrocalcinosis.

Acute flares in inflammatory arthritis

Rheumatoid arthritis and the other inflammatory arthropathies are all liable to produce acute or sub-acute flares in one or a few joints. However, there is also a small, but definite, risk in rheumatoid arthritis of pyogenic infection (p. 45). The vast majority of hip joint flares will settle over a week or so, and management by observation is therefore appropriate. However, suspicion of infection because of pyrexia, toxaemia, or worsening pain are indications for transfer to hospital for aspiration. This is carried out by passing a long needle above the greater trochanter and advancing it gently towards the gap between the femoral head and the top of the acetabular rim.

Loose fragments

In any joint a history of acute episodes of sudden painful 'locking' or 'giving way', point to the interposition of something between the bearing surfaces. Internal derangements of the knee (p. 195) are the most common cause, but loose fragments in the hip may occasionally produce a similar picture.

Referred root pains

A common diagnostic problem is the differentiation of pain arising in the lumbar spine from pain in the hip joint. The most useful method of differentiation is careful testing of hip movements. If all hip movements are full and completely painless, even at the extremes, then it is highly unlikely that the pain arises in that joint. Equally, limited and painful lumbar spine flexion and straight leg raising (p. 140) will point to a lumbar spine cause.

Psoas muscle irritation

Painful spasm of the iliopsoas muscle due to pathology in the lumbar spine or abdomen may produce an apparent flexion deformity of the hip joint. It will be found, however, that all other hip movements are full and painless.

Fractured neck of femur

Elderly osteoporotic females may fracture the neck of femur with minimal trauma. Occasionally, with an undisplaced or impacted fracture, it may even be possible for the patient to bear weight on the fractured side and to walk. In these circumstances, it is all too easy to miss the diagnosis and consider the patient to have an arthritic condition of the hip. It is essential to be aware of this possibility in patients at risk, and not to allow the patient to bear weight on the leg until a fracture has been excluded by X-ray.

Bursitis

There are a number of bursae around the hip which may occasionally become painful and mimic disease of the joint. If this diagnosis is suspected management consists of infiltrating the tender bursal site with a mixture of 2 ml hydrocortisone acetate (25 mg/ml) plus 2 ml of lignocaine (1 per cent). Dramatic relief of the pain confirms the diagnosis.

Trochanteric bursitis is the most commonly encountered. Typically there is tenderness on palpating the outermost aspect of the thigh from the top of the greater trochanter downwards for about 5 cm. In addition, pain is provoked by full adduction of the flexed hip. Other bursae which may rarely be involved are the gluteal and the ischial.

Tendinitis

Adductor tendinitis is an uncommon disorder which may result from horse riding or other types of sport. Tenderness is present over the proximal origin of the adductor muscles from the pubic ramus, and resisted adduction of the thigh provokes pain. Again, infiltration with a mixture of hydrocortisone plus lignocaine is often both diagnostic and curative.

Malignant bony deposits

Suspicion of malignant disease is likely to be aroused when hip movements are not clearly restricted, but all manipulations of the leg or pelvis produce rather widespread pains. The commonest skeletal malignancies are multiple myeloma, or secondary deposits from the bronchus, breast, or prostate.

Metabolic bone disease (see also Chapter 9)

As is the case with malignant deposits, metabolic bone disease may mimic almost any rheumatic complaint. In the case of the hip joint, osteomalacia and Paget's disease are the two bone disorders most likely to cause confusion. Serum alkaline phosphatase concentrations provide an effective screening test for both.

Causes of hip pain in children

Pain in the hip joint in a child, particularly if associated with a limp and restriction in the normal range of movements, demands careful examination, urgent review of the diagnostic possibilities and often referral for specialist investigation. Some of the conditions are listed below, together with brief notes about diagnosis.

Congenital dislocation of the hip

Failure to diagnose a dislocated hip(s) at birth leaves a child who will develop a waddling gait and positive Trendelenburg sign (p. 177). Examination reveals an increased lumbar lordosis, leg shortening and restricted abduction. The head of the femur may be palpable in the buttock, and various manoeuvres will demonstrate the 'telescoping' of the femur. X-rays are diagnostic. Girls are more commonly affected than boys (F:M = 4:1).

Slipped, upper femoral epiphysis

This uncommon condition usually presents as pain and a limp in boys aged 14–16 years or girls aged 11–13. If bilateral the gait is waddling. Examination shows movements to be limited and—highly characteristically—hip flexion produces external rotation. Initially X-rays may be negative, but will show changes if repeated after four to six weeks (lateral views are required to show the backward displacement of the epiphysis on the femoral neck). This condition may progress to aseptic necrosis of the epiphysis. Treatment is by internal fixation using pins, and occasionally intertrochanteric osteotomy. The condition has to be differentiated from Perthes' disease and from tuberculosis, in which all hip movements are more restricted.

Osteochondritis of the upper femoral epiphysis
(Legg–Calve–Perthes' disease)

Perthes' disease probably represents ischaemic necrosis of the upper femoral epiphysis. Boys are affected more often than girls (4:1) and the condition usually presents between the ages of 4 and 9 years. It is bilateral·in 15 per cent of cases. The presenting features are pain and a limp, but these may be intermittent initially. Examination shows slight reduction in internal rotation and abduction. Early X-rays may appear normal, but should be repeated after six to eight weeks. The characteristic radiological signs evolve gradually through the stages of increased density, radiolucent defects, and, finally, remodelling. These radiological changes are often more dramatic than the clinical abnormalities. Pathologically the condition is self-limiting, with more or less complete recovery over a period of two to four years. The condition is treated by rest during the active phase.

Septic arthritis (see also Chapter 8)

The hip is particularly at risk of pyogenic invasion because part of the metaphysis lies within the joint capsule. Septic arthritis usually presents dramatically and demands both immediate aspiration of the joint (under general anaesthetic if necessary) and blood culture before any antibiotics are given.

Tuberculosis (see also Chapter 8)

Any monarticular subacute arthritis must be regarded as tuberculosis until proved otherwise. In Britain the condition is most common amongst Asian immigrants. The diagnosis may require synovial biopsy (investigation of synovial fluid is frequently negative). Skeletal tuberculosis is often associated with a normal chest X-ray, but a strongly positive tuberculin skin test may provide a useful pointer.

Juvenile chronic polyarthritis

Differentiation of a monarticular onset of juvenile chronic polyarthritis in a hip joint from tuberculosis can be very difficult. In the absence of a clear radiological pointer to tuberculosis it may require open biopsy to establish the diagnosis (see above).

Haemophilia (see also Chapter 9)

Very rarely a bleed occurs into one joint in a child in whom haemophilia has not yet been diagnosed. Such a joint is excessively painful and aspiration yields pure blood.

Transient synovitis of the hip ('observation hip'; 'irritable hip')

In the early stages of most of the conditions discussed here it may be impossible to determine the cause of a painful limited hip in a child. Occasionally such a hip will resolve eventually over a period of four to six weeks, without the cause becoming apparent. The diagnostic terms above are then applied.

Spasm of the iliopsoas muscle

Spasm of the psoas in a child due to intra-abdominal conditions such as mesenteric adenitis can easily be mistaken for arthritis of the hip. Careful analysis of the physical signs should point to the correct diagnosis.

THE KNEE

The anatomy of the knee is shown in diagrammatic form in Figure 14.6. Note that the main joint compartment is at the level of the middle of the patellar ligament and that the suprapatellar pouch extends a considerable distance up the femur.

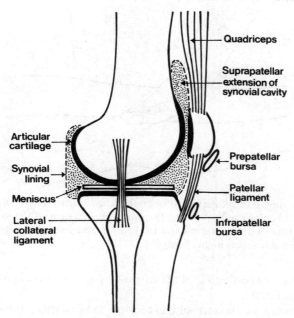

Fig. 14.6. Diagram of the anatomy of the knee joint. Note (a) that the main joint space is at the level of the middle of the patellar ligament and (b) that the synovial cavity extends for some distance upwards above the patella.

Examination of the knee

Inspect the knees with the patient lying and standing. Check the posterior (popliteal) aspect too. An effusion or thickening of the synovium shows as a bulge of the suprapatellar pouch and extends down on either side of the patella to form a horseshoe shape. Differentiating an effusion from synovial thickening requires experience. The three manoeuvres used to identify the presence of fluid are shown in Figures 2.4 (a), (b), and (c) (p. 17). The presence of an effusion is non-specific evidence of arthritis. Synovial thickening by contrast indicates an inflammatory form of synovitis (e.g. rheumatoid), while bony swelling (identified by a sensation of gnarled hard outgrowths on palpation) is evidence of osteoarthritis.

Compare the temperature of the two knee joints by placing the backs of the fingers on the patella (Fig. 14.7) and move them backwards and forwards between the two sides (but beware the joint warmed by a bandage!).

Look for wasting of the quadriceps muscles. A quick check of the state of this muscle is provided by palpating with the finger tips while the patient presses his knee down onto the couch (Fig. 2.6 p. 19). An accurate comparison between the two sides requires recording the

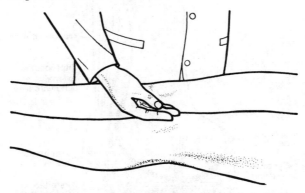

Fig. 14.7. Testing skin temperature over the knee joints. The same part of the examiner's hand (here the back of the fingers) is placed against the skin over same area of the patient's knee, and moved backwards and forwards between the two joints. This valuable test is highly sensitive.

circumference of the thigh at a set distance (e.g. 20 cm) above the upper border of the patella.

Test the range of flexion and extension movements and while doing this hold the free hand on the patella surface to feel for crepitus. This gives useful information about the state of the bearing surfaces. Note any valgus (knock-knee) or varus (bow-leg) deformity, and test for any instability (laxity) of the joint (Figs 2.5 (a) and (b) p. 18).

Careful deep palpation of the knee can be highly informative. Popliteal cysts may be identified posteriorly, while sensitive 'trigger points' may be identified in the osteoarthritic knee round the edge of the patella or round the collateral ligaments (sites where local injection of corticosteroid may be effective). Meniscal tears or cysts may be felt anteromedially or antero-laterally in the joint line if the lower leg is rotated alternately internally and externally during flexion and extension of the knee (McMurray's manoeuvre—Fig. 14.8). Irritability of the patello–femoral compartment is indicated by pain on rubbing the patella against the underlying femoral condyles, or by tipping the patella sideways and palpating the undersurface.

Clicks and cracks

A badly damaged knee may produce loud grating or clunking sounds— audible to both patient and observer—which indicate gross mechanical abnormalities. The knee may also generate loud sounds which are completely innocent. One is the loud, single 'pistol shot' sound which may occur during full knee bending under load. This represents the phenomenon of 'cavitation' in which negative pressure causes a bubble of gas to form in the synovial fluid. A similar effect can be obtained by

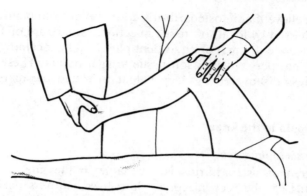

Fig. 14.8. The McMurray manoeuvre. This is a test for a torn meniscus and the same manoeuvre may be useful for freeing a knee 'locked' by a fragment of torn meniscus caught between the articulating surfaces. The knee is flexed and extended repeatedly with the tibia in different positions of internal and external rotation on the femur. The rotation is produced by the examiner's right hand grasping the sole of the foot, while the thumb of the left hand palpates the antero-medial and antero-lateral aspects of the joint line for the characteristic 'clicking' sensation of a torn meniscus or the bulge of a meniscal cyst.

hyperextension or distraction of finger joints. The other audible sound is the 'snapping' of a tendon as it slips across a prominence during flexion or extension of the knee. A palpating finger may be able to detect the movement.

Injection/aspiration of the knee joint

The knee joint is aspirated and/or injected with corticosteroid more often than any other joint in the body. The reader is strongly advised to familiarize himself both with the techniques of identifying the presence of fluid within the knee joint (p. 17) and with the method of aspirating and injecting the joint (p. 19). There are few more satisfactory means of helping the rheumatoid patient than aspirating a tense knee effusion and then replacing this with a small volume of corticosteroid suspension.

The anti-inflammatory effects of intra-articular steroid injections last days, weeks, or sometimes months, and the question therefore arises as to how often they should be repeated. In the past fears have been expressed that repeated injections may lead to destructive changes in the joint. Very extensive experience now suggests that this is not the case (Hollander 1985) and there seems no point in denying one's patients the benefit of three or four such injections per year—if these provide good symptomatic relief.

Apart from injecting corticosteroids directly into the knee joint, some clinicians believe that in osteoarthritis useful relief from painful episodes may be achieved by local soft tissue injections. A mixture of 1 ml hydrocortisone acetate (25 mg) or equivalent plus 1 ml lignocaine (1 per cent) is injected into peri-articular soft tissue 'trigger points'. These are points of tenderness discovered by deep palpation round the margins of the joint.

Causes of pain in the knee

Osteoarthritis of the knee

Some degree of osteoarthritis is invariable in the knees of the very elderly. This can be recognized by short-lived stiffness ('gelling') after periods of immobility, the presence of palpable osteophytes, crepitus on movement, and sometimes small effusions. So long as some thickness of cartilage remains on the bearing surfaces, and the muscles acting across the knees are strong enough to maintain stability and alignment, this does not cause much problem. Such patients need to be advised to carry out a daily 'quadriceps drill', to use their knees for weight-bearing only when they need to do so, and to use a walking stick in the opposite hand if and when they go through a more painful patch. If they are unsteady on their legs they should always use a stick.

The more difficult problem is the middle-aged or older patient—more often a woman—in whom progressive knee osteoarthritis is associated with obesity, flabby muscles and progressive instability of the knees. Such patients may cope with the problem so long as the alignment of the knees remains normal, but once collapse of the medial tibial plateau produces a varus (bow leg) deformity (or, less often, collapse of the lateral side produces genu valgum—knock-knee) then pain and disability often become rapidly progressive. The changes in the main knee compartment and the patello–femoral compartment may be affected to different degrees. Pain on negotiating stairs and on rising from a chair are features which point particularly to patello–femoral involvement. Weight-bearing X-rays provide a good assessment of the state of such joints.

Conservative treatment has little to offer such patients. Weight reduction usually proves an elusive goal, while muscle strengthening by active, resisted exercises—although always aimed for—requires considerable dedication to achieve results. Analgesics and anti-inflammatory drugs are prescribed, but generally achieve less than in more 'inflammatory' conditions. The only splint likely to be of value is the 'telescopic' Canadian (CARS-B) splint which in theory can counteract the tendency to varus or valgus deformity while allowing flexion and extension movements. Unfortunately, it is often not effective when used for obese legs. Intra-articular injections of corticosteroid may occasionally be useful in tiding the patient over a bad patch. It may also be worth injecting a tender peri-articular trigger point (p. 12).

The single most useful conservative measure is the use of a walking stick in the hand opposite the bad knee. The stick must be of correct length (p. 181) and it is usually advisable for the patient to be instructed in its use by a physiotherapist. Some patients may require two sticks or a quadripod. Vanity often makes patients try and manage without a stick.

Surgery provides the long-stop for those whose general health allows it. Particularly if only one knee is affected the result can be highly successful. An essential objective is to correct alignment. This can be achieved by double (above and below) or single osteotomy, or correcting alignment can be combined with resurfacing the joint by total replacement.

Rheumatoid arthritis (and other inflammatory arthropathies) of the knee joint (see also Chapters 3 and 4)

Involvement of the knees is the most common reason for a patient with rheumatoid (or other inflammatory arthropathy) to take to a wheelchair. Despite the most conscientious application of the management measures outlined in Chapter 3 (second-line drugs, muscle-strengthening exercises, occasional intra-articular corticosteroid injections, etc.) some rheumatoid patients' knees deteriorate inexorably to a point where valgus (knock-knee) and flexion deformities finally make walking impossible. Much can be done to maintain partial mobility by the use of appropriate walking aids, including walking frames, if necessary fitted with forearm rests. At this stage the patient needs to be in touch with a hospital department of physiotherapy and occupational therapy.

The question of surgery is discussed above in connection with the hip. For the rheumatoid patient with damage in a single, large, lower limb joint, total prosthetic replacement can work a miracle. However, the more joints that will need surgery, the more daunting becomes the prospect. The remarks above relating to the use of the Canadian splint for varus deformities of osteoarthritis apply also to the common rheumatoid valgus deformity.

Chondromalacia patellae (anterior knee pain)

This term is applied to a painful knee condition seen most commonly in teenagers or young adults, often rather athletic females. The typical history is of a dull ache behind the patella of one or both knees coming on during and after physical activity such as ball games at school. Pain on negotiating stairs may point to involvement of the patello–femoral compartment.

On examination the knee is cool and rarely contains an effusion. The range of normal knee movements is full and any quadriceps wasting is modest. The positive physical signs consist of pain on pressing or rubbing the patella againts the underlying femoral condyles (particularly during contraction of the quadriceps). The patella (sometimes unusually mobile) when tipped to one side is tender on the undersurface.

The aetiology and pathology are not known. In severe cases the cartilage on the undersurface of the patella udergoes changes similar to those of early osteoarthritis. Some believe that altered geometry of the patello–femoral bearing surfaces may play a role in causing the condition.

Fortunately the condition is self-limiting and most of these patients recover spontaneously over a period of months or years. The accepted advice is to rest the knee and to avoid all activities which bring on the pain. Predictably, in athletic young girls, this can lead to frustration and dissatisfaction with the lack of more positive treatment. Quadriceps drill is usually prescribed, and sometimes other forms of physiotherapy, but there is no evidence that this does any more than satisfy the patient and her family that 'something is being done' while nature takes its course. The same is probably true of the various operations such as cartilage shaving or drilling which are sometimes undertaken in the most resistant cases.

Fortunately most patients eventually make a complete or near-complete recovery and late residual disability appears to be uncommon.

Bursitis

The two bursae in front of and at the lower border of the patella (pre-patellar and infra-patellar—Fig. 14.6) are liable to inflammation. Chronic kneeling trauma may produce low-grade inflammatory changes with chronic effusions. If such lesions are troublesome the bursa in question can be excised.

More active inflammatory changes can be painful and make kneeling difficult, in which case a local injection of corticosteroid may settle the inflammation.

Pyogenic infection of the bursae produces an extremely acute inflammatory picture with severe pain, redness, and spreading cellulitis of surrounding tissues. This lesion may easily be mistaken for septic arthritis of the knee joint. Management consists of intensive antibiotic treatment. Surgical drainage is seldom necessary.

Osteochondritis dissecans

Occasionally a piece of articular cartilage, perhaps 0.5–1.5 cm in diameter, becomes separated from one of the femoral condyles. It may carry some underlying bone with it. The separated material then lies free in the synovial fluid as a loose body. If and when it gets caught between the articular surfaces it will produce the characteristic symptoms of a loose body: 'locking' or 'giving way', associated with pain, and usually followed by an effusion lasting a few days. X-rays will show the fragment if there is bone attached and the bony defect in the femoral condyle may be visible. Treatment is removal, either endoscopically or by open arthrotomy.

Osteochondromatosis

For reasons which are not understood, the synovium of the knee occasionally undergoes metaplasia to cartilage and bone. These pedunculated lobules of material are then liable to become caught between the articular surfaces to produce 'locking' or 'giving way', as in the case of osteochondritis dissecans (see above). X-rays reveal a calcified 'bunch of grapes'. Treatment is by surgical excision (synovectomy) of the abnormal tissue.

Synovial rupture and Baker's cysts

Within the normal knee synovial fluid is at approximately atmospheric pressure. As the volume of fluid increases with an effusion, so this pressure rises until, during violent flexion movement, peak pressures equal to arterial blood pressure may develop. It is under these circumstances that the synovial cavity may rupture. This happens most often in the rheumatoid knee, but effusions from any cause may produce a rupture.

Ruptures invariably occur posteriorly, and the most dramatic outcome is for the fluid to track down into the calf muscles. Occasionally the patient will describe how sudden calf pain and swelling developed at the same time as the knee swelling disappeared. Examination reveals a tender, swollen, warm calf, sometimes with overlying erythema, and a positive Homans' sign (calf pain and resistance on forced dorsiflexion of the foot with the knee extended). In other words the physical signs closely mimic those of calf vein thrombosis. The differentiation is clearly critical from the management point of view. Intra-articular injection of radio-opaque dye followed by exercising the joint will show dye tracking into the calf. However, the more important issue is to exclude a venous thrombosis, so venography is usually the preferred investigation.

Rarely a cystic swelling may persist in the calf (and occasionally require surgical removal); more often the calf signs resolve uneventfully. However, a tense cystic swelling may be left in the popliteal fossa (Baker's cyst). Alternatively, such a cyst may develop gradually without a frank rupture being recognized. Such popliteal cysts can be a major cause of discomfort in the rheumatoid knee. To the observer they feel like hard bantam-egg-sized swellings in the popliteal fossa.

It is thought that popliteal cysts form following a posterior rupture. A track develops between the joint cavity and the cyst which includes a valve mechanism such that joint movements cause fluid to be pumped from the joint into the cyst. Fluid can escape from the cyst only by ultra-filtration into the surrounding tissues, a process which leaves the larger fibrinogen molecules behind. The cyst thus comes to contain fibrinogen and fluid with a high protein content. It is tense and tends to grow gradually.

Treatment is difficult. Excision of the cyst is technically complicated and is likely to be followed by recurrence. The most hopeful approach seems to be to try and 'dry up' the source of the fluid either by intra-articular corticosteroid injection or by surgical synovectomy.

Traumatic knee problems

Ligamentous injuries

Ligamentous injuries to the knee are difficult to diagnose. This history is often misleading and the signs frequently deceptive (Apley and Solomon 1982). The commonest causes are sports injuries and traffic accidents, in both of which the history of the injury may be confused. Further, partial ligamentous tears may produce more obvious signs than complete tears, which are often missed.

On initial examination bruising may indicate the site of ligamentous damage. On stressing the various ligaments, partial tears permit no abnormal movement, but the attempt causes local pain. Complete tears allow abnormal movements which, deceptively, may be painless. The treatment of these two conditions is different and, if necessary, the joint may need to be examined under an anaesthetic.

Three planes of movement must be tested in order to identify a complete ligamentous tear:

1. Sideways tilting with the knee in full extension and in partial flexion up to 30° Fig. 2.5.A p. 18).
2. Anteroposterior gliding movements (Fig. 2.5.B p. 18).
3. Internal and external rotation of the lower leg on the femur with the knee flexed to 60°–90°.

Any definite increase in the range of any of these movements compared with the other side is an indication for operation. X-rays may show avulsion of a small piece of bone attached to a collateral or cruciate ligament. Abnormal movements may also be confirmed by X-rays of the stressed knee.

Partial tears are treated by a padded bandage, active physiotherapy, local anaesthetic injections, and aspiration of effusions. Complete tears require operative repair as early as possible, certainly within two weeks. Many general practitioners will wish to seek a specialist consultation early unless they are confident that there is no complete ligament tear and the pain improves soon after the injury.

Meniscal lesions

The medial meniscus is more often damaged than the lateral. The cause is usually a twisting strain on a partially flexed, weight-bearing knee, as when a footballer kicks across his line of running.

A careful history is critical in making a correct diagnosis. In a footballer there is immediate pain over the (usually) medial side of the joint line, sometimes 'locking' (inability to extend the joint) and, within a few hours, swelling. After two or three days there may be apparent complete recovery. After the age of 40 years the original injury may be missed. Following this there are recurrent episodes of 'locking', 'giving way', medial pain, or clicking, followed by transient swelling. Between attacks McMurray's test may be positive (Fig. 14.8). The presence of a meniscal tear may be confirmed by arthrography (ideally with liquid/gas double contrast) or arthroscopy. Conservative treatment (splinting, followed by physiotherapy and avoidance of precipitating factors) may occasionally be adequate. Recurrent episodes demand operative treatment. Lateral meniscal lesions are much less common but may occasionally require meniscal excision.

Traumatic haemarthrosis

Any significant effusion following trauma requires aspiration. If this yields blood, then it becomes essential to examine the joint very carefully to check for ligamentous damage (see above) and to X-ray the knees (both!) to check for an avulsion or other fracture.

REFERENCES

Adams, J. C. (1981). Hip region. In *Outline of orthopaedics*, (9th edn). (Chapter 8, pp. 311–61). Churchill Livingstone, London.
Apley, A. G. and Solomon, L. (1982). Knee ligament injuries. In *Apley's system of orthopaedics and fractures*, (6th edn) (pp. 456–9). Butterworth, London.

15 Regional problems VI:

The ankle and foot

Functional anatomy

The ankle joint is a simple mortice, the talus being held between the tibia and fibula, and depends on a series of medial and lateral ligaments for its integrity (Fig. 15.2). The ankle joint allows only two movements; plantar flexion is served by the gastrocnemius and soleus, assisted by the long flexors of the toes, dorsiflexion by the tibialis anterior assisted by the long extensors of the toes. The subtalar joint separates the talus from the

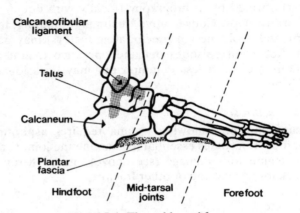

Fig. 15.1. The ankle and foot.

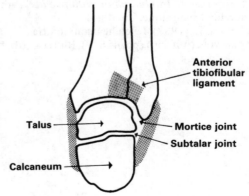

Fig. 15.2. The mortice joint at the ankle.

196

calcaneum, which forms the heel. This joint is commonly affected by both osteoarthritis and rheumatoid arthritis. The talus and calcaneum articulate with the small tarsal bones to form the mid-tarsal joints, which allow circumduction of the forefoot. The metatarsophalangeal joints allow rotational movement (similar to the metacarpophalangeal joints), and the interphalangeal joints are hinges. When examining for tenderness and range of movement at these joints the best comparison is with the joints of the other foot, as there is considerable normal variation between people's feet.

DISORDERS OF THE LOWER LEG, ANKLE, AND HEEL

Torn gastrocnemius muscle (tennis leg)

The history in this condition is characteristic. The patient reports that he was walking briskly when he suddenly experienced acute pain behind the knee as though hit with something; from then on walking is limited to hobbling on tiptoe. Examination shows tenderness in the calf. Resisted plantar flexion should be tested with the patient lying prone; it will be found to be painful when the knee is extended (gastrocnemius action), but pain free when the knee is flexed to 90 degrees (soleus action). Treatment includes rest, a heel raise to prevent painful extension of the muscle, a stick, and non-weight-bearing exercises—moving the foot up and down while lying down. Ultrasound and heat treatment from a physiotherapist may also give transient pain relief. If there is a bad tear it may be three or four weeks before the patient can stand on tiptoe painlessly.

Sprained ankle

The commonest cause of a sprained ankle is an inversion injury of the foot, causing a partial tear of the lateral calcaneo-fibular ligament (Fig. 15.1). A sprained ankle can be treated in the surgery if the ankle joint is stable, that is if there are no fractures and the ligaments holding the mortice joint have not been ruptured. The stability of the mortice can be tested by gentle traction of the foot with the ankle at 90 degrees, and by inversion and eversion of the ankle. The range should be compared with the normal side. Pain and swelling often make interpretation of these signs difficult. If doubt exists a specialist opinion should be sought, as a neglected rupture of the lateral ligament can lead to persistent instability.

Management

A firm bandage is applied from the toes to the mid-calf. The foot is elevated, and ice packs applied, these act as an analgesic and may limit the oedema. Early mobilizing exercises are begun the next day, non-weight-bearing if necessary. A moderately severe sprain will take two or three weeks before walking is comfortable. Vigorous exercise will not be safe for about three months after a bad sprain. Patients are often surprised at the length of time recovery takes, so it is important to stress this early on and also that the foot will have a tendency to swell for many months afterwards. If physiotherapy is requested or required, ultrasound to the damaged ligament and supervised exercise are usually prescribed.

Achilles' tendinitis and bursitis

A ruptured Achilles' tendon is demonstrated by the inability to stand on the toes of the affected foot. Palpation reveals a gap in the tendon. This injury will need either immediate surgical repair or immobilization in plaster, and should be referred the same day. Inflammation can occur at the insertion of the tendon into the calcaneum, causing pain in the posterior part of the heel on walking. Inflammation can also occur along the length of the tendon or in the bursa which lies between it and the calcaneum (Fig. 15.3). In this condition the patient reports pain after walking and exercise, or a poorly localized ache above the heel. Treatment can involve immobilization to await natural resolution, or infiltration with a steroid preparation into the painful site. It is important to avoid injecting directly into the tendon as it is thought this predisposes to rupture.

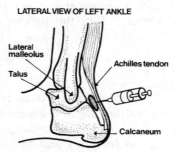

LATERAL VIEW OF LEFT ANKLE

Lateral malleolus

Talus

Achilles tendon

Calcaneum

Fig. 15.3. Injection site for Achilles' tendinitis and bursitis.

Plantar fasciitis

The plantar fascia runs from the calcaneum to the base of the toes. It is part of the soft tissue bridge which maintains the longitudinal arch of the foot. A strain or tear at the calcaneal insertion may produce a bony spur as the periosteum is pulled away from the bone. Painless spurs are quite frequent X-ray findings and are of no significance. Painful plantar fasciitis may develop with or without the formation of a spur, it may

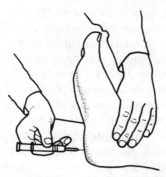

Fig. 15.4. Injection technique for plantar fasciitis.

complicate the course of one of the seronegative arthropathies, and this should be suspected if X-rays of the heel show an eroded, irregular or fluffy calcaneal spur. Whatever the cause, the patient will describe pain deep in the heel. It is commonly worst when the patient first gets out of bed, and persists as a dull ache all day. Treatment is aimed at relieving the inflammation and taking the strain off the plantar fascia. A local steroid injection often gives relief. Using a 23 gauge (blue) needle and the usual aseptic technique, the injection is placed in the centre of the plantar surface of the heel at the site of maximum tenderness. The needle is inserted until resistance is met, and then withdrawn a little before the injection is given (Fig. 15.4).

A rubber heel 'shock absorber' placed inside the shoe redistributes the pattern of weight-bearing in the foot and diminishes the stretch in the plantar fascia. This may give considerable pain relief. Resistant cases are sometimes helped by ultrasound.

Tarsal tunnel syndrome

This is an uncommon nerve-entrapment syndrome which parallels the carpal tunnel syndrome at the wrist. The posterior tibial nerve is compressed as it runs under the flexor retinaculum, behind the medial malleolus. The patient complains of pain, numbness or tingling along the medial border of the foot and the first toe. Treatment is by surgical decompression.

INFLAMMATORY ARTHRITIS AT THE ANKLE AND MID-TARSAL JOINTS

The mortice joint at the ankle is a less common site for inflammatory arthritis than the sub-talar joint which may be severely affected by rheumatoid arthritis, giving rise to pain in the hindfoot on walking. The seronegative forms of arthritis such as Reiter's and psoriatic arthritis may also affect the small mid-tarsal joints of the foot. The joints will be painful, warm and have a restricted range of movement. Arthritis at the sub-talar and mid-tarsal joints can have serious consequences. As the destructive, inflammatory process develops the bony surfaces of the joints are destroyed and the ligaments become lax. Eventually the joints become unstable and subluxation occurs. Owing to the weight-bearing involved in walking the mid- and hind-foot become progressively deformed. The ankle usually develops a valgus deformity and the longitudinal arch becomes flattened (Fig. 3.7). Treatment of the general condition should proceed along the usual lines (see Chapters 3 and 4). Specific treatment includes:

> Referral to the occupational therapist to get advice on appropriate footwear. This may involve getting custom-built shoes, or thermo-plastic moulded footwear (Drushoes).
> A lightweight fibreglass heelcup, worn inside the shoe which helps to prevent further valgus deformity at the ankle.
> Arthrodesis to fixate the joints.

THE FOREFOOT

Metatarsalgia is the term used to describe forefoot pain. There are many different causes (described below, and in Fig. 15.5), but the common feature is an alteration in the weight-bearing pattern at the metatarsal heads. Patients may describe their symptoms simply as an ache in the foot towards the end of the day, or as a burning sensation in the sole of the foot. If the metatarsal heads are not well aligned on the fibro-fatty pad which normally acts as a shock absorber, symptoms may be likened to walking on pebbles. Although some foot problems may seem relatively minor to the doctor, there is no doubt that many elderly people become housebound due to problems with their feet which may be eminently treatable.

Causes of metatarsalgia

Fibro-fatty pad degeneration

This is a common complaint amongst the elderly, and is made worse by conditions associated with vascular insufficiency, where there is thinning of tissues and poor nutrition of the feet. Treatment involves making an insole which takes the weight off the metatarsal heads, or fitting a metatarsal bar to the sole of the shoe which redistributes the main body weight to a point just behind the metatarsal heads.

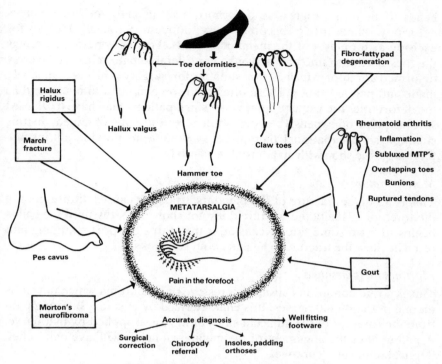

Fig. 15.5. Some of the causes of metatarsalgia.

Rheumatoid arthritis

The metatarsophalangeal joints are commonly affected early in the course of this disease. Pain and swelling widens the forefoot and makes shoe fitting difficult. Erosive destruction of the heads of the metatarsophalangeal joints coupled with the ligamentous laxity which follows repeated swelling of the joint capsule, causes subluxation. This may occur vertically to form the claw toe deformity, or laterally to form a progressive valgus deformity of the toes. If it is left uncorrected the patient will develop overriding toes, painful interdigital corns, fungal infections, and bunions over the first and fifth metatarsophalangeal joints. Problems at the forefoot may be compounded by inflammatory damage at the subtalar joint of the heel, and by vasculitis causing ulceration. For a patient with arthritis of the knees and hands it may be the development of foot problems that confines her to her home or a wheelchair.

Early treatment of the rheumatoid forefoot involves advice about footwear—square toes, low heel, a fastening that allows for widening of the forefoot, and an insole to take the weight off the painful metatarsal heads. If there is progressive deformity, such as claw toes or a valgus deformity, shoe fitting becomes very difficult. Surgical referral for excision arthroplasty of the metatarsal heads (Fowler's operation) brings the toes back into line and may give considerable pain relief. A severely deformed forefoot which is not suitable for surgery will need specially made and padded shoes. These often take some months to make, and as the deformities are usually progressive some patients may have to discard several pairs of expensive shoes soon after they are obtained. In this situation an occupational therapist may be able to provide an 'instant' thermoplastic shoe with an adjustable velcro fastening.

March fracture

This is a fatigue fracture of the metatarsal shaft. It causes diffuse pain in the forefoot. Usually the fracture does not show on X-ray until the callus begins to form some three weeks after the injury. Support strapping and rest will allow the fracture to heal in about six weeks.

Morton's metatarsalgia

This is a rare condition caused by pressure on a neuroma which develops on one of the digital nerves. It is characterized by episodic shooting pain from the forefoot to the adjacent sides of the toes supplied by that nerve. A pad to alter the alignment of the metatarsal heads will give pain relief. Surgical removal is curative.

Hallux rigidus

This is osteoarthritis at the first metatarsophalangeal joint and may follow osteochondritis of the metatarsal in adolescence. The great toe is painful on extension, which occurs every time the patient takes a step. Stiffening the sole of the shoe or providing a 'rocker' sole can alleviate symptoms. Surgical fusion of the joint may be necessary in severe cases.

Toe deformities

Shoes which are too short or too pointed cause impaction or bunching of the toes. In time this develops into hammer toe and claw toe deformities which produce problems with shoe fitting and are frequently the site of painful corns. As the toes do not participate equally in weight-bearing they cause back pressure and overloading on the metatarsophalangeal joints, and eventually metatarsalgia. If very troublesome the toes may need surgical straightening, and the sole of the foot a metatarsal support pad to relieve the metatarsalgia. Hallux valgus also causes shoe fitting problems. If wide, square-toed shoes are not worn, interdigital corns and bunions develop from the continuous pressure and friction. A bunion is bursitis at the medial aspect of the head of the first metatarsal (small bunions, bunionettes, may also develop on the lateral aspect of the fifth metatarsal). An excision arthroplasty of the first metatarsophalangeal joint (Keller's operation) straightens the great toe and allows normal shoes to be worn in comfort.

Gout

The first metatarsophalangeal joint is affected by gout in about 75 per cent of attacks. The joint is red, hot, and very tender. The acute attack settles rapidly with indomethacin, but the condition should be further investigated (see Chapter 5).

Other foot deformities

Pes cavus, a high, arched foot with claw toes, commonly results in metatarsalgia as the metatarsophalangeal joints are overloaded. It may occur sporadically or in combination with neurological conditions such as Friedrich's ataxia, spina bifida, and peroneal muscular atrophy. Special shoes may be needed with an insole to redistribute the load over the whole foot.

CHILDREN'S FEET

General practitioners, especially those who run well baby clinics, are frequently consulted about a number of minor structural variations in babies' and toddlers' feet. The foot of a normal baby is very mobile: plantar flexion should align the toes in a continuous straight line with the tibia, dorsiflexion should allow the dorsum of the foot to touch the front of the leg. This mobility is absent in the various forms of club foot, which all need early management by an orthopaedic surgeon.

The toddler's foot is chubby, and is flat because of the normal plantar fat pad which gradually diminishes between the ages of 2 and 3 years. Most infants have bow legs due to curving of the tibia. As the child learns to walk this usually changes to a knock-knee posture, which deteriorates until the child is about 3 years old and then begins to straighten, usually disappearing by the age of 7. Knock-knees and bow legs at this age only need further investigation if there is asymmetry of the deformity (e.g. rickety bow legs). If a knock-knee deformity is increasing after the age of 5 or 6 years (if the distance between the medial malleoli of the ankles is greater than 10 cm with the child lying down with the knees together) then referral is indicated, although surgical correction is rarely required.

In-toeing gait (pigeon toes)

An in-toeing gait may be due to the foot, tibia, or femur. The great majority cause no significant disability.

Hooked forefoot (adducted forefoot)

In this condition the front part of the foot turns inwards but the heel is normal (Fig. 15.6). In the normal foot a line drawn through the centre of the heel should run between the second and third toe. In the adducted forefoot it runs further laterally.

This condition poses considerable difficulties in shoe fitting and can be easily corrected by splinting in infancy, so it is worth referring patients early.

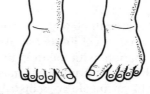

Fig. 15.6. The adducted forefoot.

Tibial torsion

Most mild degrees of in-toeing occur because there is internal torsion of the tibia (Fig. 15.7 (a)). When the child stands, the patellae point forward but the feet point inwards. The condition resolves spontaneously as the tibia de-rotates during growth.

Femoral neck anteversion

If there is a significant degree of femoral anteversion the whole leg will turn inwards (Fig. 15.7 (b)). On examining the child standing it will be seen that, as well as the feet in-turning, the patellae face inwards rather than forwards (squinting patellae). Examination with the child lying supine will show a greater than normal range of internal rotation at the hips and a loss of external rotation (normally they are about equal). Most children with femoral anteversion develop a compensatory external tibial torsion which straightens the feet in time. If there is severe in-toeing with squinting patellae which persists into the seventh or eighth year, referral should be considered, although a corrective osteotomy is very rarely necessary.

Flat feet

Flat feet are normal in infancy. Parents often worry about them in young children, but if they are pain free and mobile (can the child stand on tiptoes?) they are a normal variant and need no special treatment or exercise regimen.

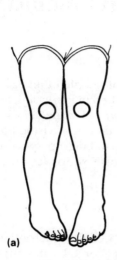 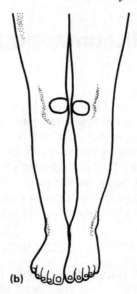

(a)   (b)

Fig. 15.7(a). In-toeing as a result of tibial torsion.
15.7(b). Persistent femoral anteversion and squinting patellae.

Children's shoes

When patients show concern about their children's feet it is a good opportunity to give advice on footwear. A growing foot is very easily compressed and moulded. The common problems are shoes *and socks* that are too small, or long, loose shoes that allow forward slip and impaction of the toes. Girls' pointed shoes are a potent cause of hallux valgus; by the age of 8 years differences in the appearances of boys' and girls' feet can already be seen. Toe deformities cause corns and calluses, and are a cause of metatarsalgia in later life.

REFERENCES

Cyriax, J. (1982). *Textbook of orthopaedic medicine*. Vol. 1 (8th edn). Balliere Tindall, London.

Dixon, A. StJ. The rheumatoid foot. In *Rheumatic diseases: Collected reports 1959–1983*. Arthritis and Rheumatism Council, London.

Jayson, M. and Million, R. (eds) (1983). *Locomotor disorders in general practice*. Oxford University Press, Oxford.

Neale, D. (ed.) (1981). *Common foot disorders: diagnosis and management*. Churchill Livingstone, London.

16 Rheumatology in sports medicine

There has been an explosion in the numbers of people of all ages taking up physical sports for recreation. This has resulted in increasing demands on general practitioners for involvement in all aspects of 'sports medicine'. The practitioner's role ranges from that of advising about the value of 'keep-fit' exercises or the question of taking up sport again in middle age, to the management of minor 'overuse' sports lesions, as well as dealing with more urgent acute injuries.

THE SPORTS INJURY CLINIC

Many hospitals now provide open access to a clinic which offers early investigation and treatment of sports injuries. For GPs this provides a convenient means of getting early diagnostic and management advice, and of obtaining early physiotherapy for patients with recent injuries. Staff working together in such clinics develop management strategies which can make the most effective and economical use of available resources.

ADVICE ABOUT 'KEEP-FIT' ACTIVITIES

Despite the views of the lay public, the medical advantages of 'keeping fit' by taking regular exercise—over and above normal daily activities—are not well established. There is evidence that the inevitable loss of bone in older subjects is slowed by the pull of muscles on the skeleton: equally it is common experience that regular physical exercise gives a sense of both physical and psychological well-being. However, lack of exercise does not rank as a health hazard in the same way that obesity or smoking and alcohol excess do, and patients unable to take regular exercise can be reassured about this.

It is advisable to question the over-40s who seek advice on taking up jogging or some similar activity about chest pain and other cardiac symptoms, and to check their blood pressure and urine. Judgement is needed, for example, in advising about such activities in a man with atypical chest pain. Physical activity should be stopped in the face of increasing chest pain. There is much to be said for those in middle age contemplating taking up a 'keep-fit' activity joining an appropriate club. This should provide the opportunity for getting expert advice on matters such as equipment (particularly footwear) and the grading of activities to take account of age, build, and state of fitness. Most subjects can learn to measure their own pulse rates, and this can be a useful means of monitoring progress in a programme of keep-fit activities. Exercises should not be continued beyond the point at which the pulse rate reaches 70 per cent of the maximum for the age of the subject (Table 16.1). Particular emphasis should be placed on the importance of correct footwear. Recent years have seen important advances in the understanding of the type of footwear best suited for activities such as jogging. Sperryn (1983) lists the desirable features as:

Toe area wide and rounded.
One to two layers of resiliant soling.
Hardwearing outer sole with good grip, curved round and upwards at the toe and heel.
One piece toe boxing with side reinforcement.
Heel raised and reinforced at sides.
Low back, no tab.
Minimum cushioning at the collar.
Short laces.

Those taking up new sporting activities may consult their GPs about familiar muscular problems such as stiffness and cramps. *Muscle stiffness* following exercise occurs because the unaccustomed activity produces increased capillary leakage of fluid into the extracellular compartment of the muscle. The resulting increase in intramuscular pressure accounts for the stiffness and pain on contraction. Such stiffness is evidence of the subject being 'unfit' and indicates the need for grading training activities. In one site—the anterior compartment of the lower leg—this type of muscle swelling may have serious consequences (because of the unyielding nature of the surrounding tissues). Pain persisting for hours, swelling, tenderness, redness, and oedema are indications for referral to

Table 16.1. *Mean heart rates for men and women of different ages during maximum exercise. Seventy per cent values are also shown. Data derived from Astrand and Rodahl (1977)*

Age	Maximum exercise heart rate	70 per cent value
20	200	140
30	187	131
40	180	126
50	172	120
60	160	112

hospital for consideration of surgical decompression. The outcome of this 'anterior tibial syndrome' may exceptionally be either muscle necrosis or contracture. *Muscle cramps* can be extremely distressing in older patients who have taken unaccustomed exercise. They represent an exaggeration of the spontaneous nocturnal cramps to which older subjects are liable. They commonly occur at night, in bed, and result from lowering of the neuromuscular excitability threshold. Strong muscle contractions (as in stretching the legs in bed) may set off the cramps, and sufferers may learn to avoid these. However, an attack may be terminated by actively contracting the opposing muscle, or by standing out of bed if a calf muscle is affected. A generally effective form of prevention is to raise the neuromusclar threshold by an evening dose of quinine 300 mg.

EXERCISES FOR PATIENTS WITH ARTHRITIS

Patients suffering from arthritis require advice about how much exercise and physical activity they should undertake. Generally it is safe to advise them to keep active to whatever extent they feel inclined, and to point out that activities within the pain-free range are unlikely to be harmful to joints. Patients suffering from ankylosing spondylitis need to be indoctrinated about the need for regular physical exercise (see p. 56), while those with poor quadriceps function due to arthritis of a knee joint should follow a regular routine of active, resisted exercises. However, this latter form of exercise, is more in the realm of remedial physiotherapy than 'sport'. Those with polyarticular disease (such as rheumatoid arthritis) should be advised to take whatever exercise they can within their pain-free limits. Such patients are usually restricted by pain in the legs, and it is sensible to suggest that they should consider non-weight-bearing activities such as swimming or bicycling. Some public swimming pools offer special facilities and help for the physically handicapped. Those who have recently undergone surgery, or who require strict rest, need a physiotherapist to instruct them in exercises which maintain general fitness but do not stress vulnerable joints.

TRAINING FOR SPORT

Munrow (1962) classifies the various components of training into:

1. Strength.
2. Endurance, subdivided into:
   (a) local muscular endurance;
   (b) circulo-respiratory endurance;
   (c) expedition-type endurance.
3. Mobility.
4. Skill.

Successful training for different sports requires varying proportions of these elements. The subject lies more in the realm of coaching than sports medicine. However, effective training is an essential element in the prevention of sports injuries. Indeed it is important to appreciate that most sports injuries occur outside competition and represent overuse lesions or strains, rather than trauma. The principles employed are thus applicable to less formal keep-fit activities. These include the grading and build-up of physical activities as fitness improves, and a regular routine of simple stretching and warm-up exercises to be performed before starting a game.

OVERUSE INJURIES

Overuse injuries are generally related to training, particularly doing repetitive manoeuvres incorrectly and/or too often. The first line of treatment is to change the particular technique or to use an alternative training method until the lesion is healed. Local corticosteroid injections may produce a local anti-inflammatory effect. It goes without saying that prevention is better than treatment; hence the importance of expert advice about both techniques and equipment when taking up a new sport.

In the case of many overuse injuries both the cause and the treatment is self-evident to the person concerned; for example, the oarsman's blistered hand or the jogger's raw toe. More likely to reach the attention of the general practitioner are the various forms of tendinitis, in which excessive use of a particular muscle produces mechanical irritation between the tendon and the surrounding sheath or other soft tissues. Typical examples are supraspinatus tendinitis at the shoulder (see p. 161) and Achilles' tendinitis at the heel (p. 198). These are both discussed in other sections of this book. Here it is necessary only to draw attention again to the importance of the general practitioner learning the techniques of local corticosteroid injections in order to provide early treatment. Equally important is the need to seek out and eliminate the cause in order to prevent recurrence. Enthesopathies such as tennis elbow may be particularly troublesome in this regard. Relapses on returning to playing may be prevented by adjusting technique or wearing a forearm 'Medisplint' or strapping.

ACUTE INJURIES

Acute sports injuries may result either from strains or tearing of tissues, or from direct trauma. Unlike overuse injuries, strains and tearing injuries usually result either from doing an unusual manoeuvre not trained for, or from making a maximum effort when muscles are tired and less co-ordinated than usual. The immediate mechanical cause typically relates to agonist/antagnoist muscle imbalance.

Acute sports injuries may involve muscles, tendons, bones, joints or other structures. The more serious may require specialist managment in hospital, but the majority can be managed by the general practitioner. The initial—first aid—treatment of soft tissue injuries is simple, but important and much neglected. The standard management is the R.I.C.E. method:

Rest.
Ice.
Compression.
Elevation.

This certainly provides pain relief. It may contribute to reducing inflammation. Physiotherapy methods play an important part in early treatment and, for simple injuries, much can be done by do-it-yourself techniques at home. Experience shows that cooling is most effective during the first forty-eight hours. At home this can be achieved, for example, by the application for twenty minutes at a time of a packet of frozen peas wrapped in a towel. Later, heat (in the form of a hot water bottle) can be helpful in relieving pain and assisting with gentle mobiliza- tion. Next, specific exercises for the injured area are started—always using a grade programme adjusted to the progress of recovery (indicated mainly by the level of pain). Keen sportsmen may require to be reminded that heroic efforts in the face of pain are likely to be counterproductive.

A useful measure is to start the injured person on a programme of 'alternative training'. For example, someone with a calf strain can be prescribed a programme of weight training, swimming, and even riding a bicycle—provided he keeps only his heels on the pedals. Such activities allow aerobic fitness to be maintained during the period that the carefully graded physiotherapy for the injured calf is being introduced. In this way, once the injured part is ready for a return to sport, the patient is also generally fit for this.

Tendon injuries

Tendon rupture

This is most common in those aged over 40 years, and it is likely that central degeneration plays a role. Complete rupture generally occurs abruptly without warning during strenuous activity. Rarely, direct trauma may be responsible. The diagnosis is usually made on the basis of abnormal bulging of the muscle concerned, an obvious gap in the tendon, and/or loss of the active movement subserved by the tendon (with a full range of passive movement). Ruptured tendons can be managed conservatively. However, most authorities favour immediate suture. Cases of complete rupture should therefore be referred immediately for consideration of suture.

Partial rupture

This results from the same cause as complete rupture. The signs of loss of continuity are absent, but the patient complains of local pain and stiffness on rising in the morning and on undertaking exercise. Physical examination reveals local tenderness with or without some swelling of the tendon. Treatment consists of initial rest, followed by graded activity. Physiotherapy (e.g. ultrasound) is often prescribed, but its value is unproven. In chronic and persistent cases, in which degeneration is suspected, it may be necessary to explore the lesion surgically. Local injection of corticosteroid around tendons may be undertaken if there appears to be 'peri-tendinitis'. However, corticosteroid injections into the substance of tendons are avoided as these are thought to predispose to rupture.

Muscle injuries

Complete rupture of a muscle is rare. More common is partial rupture ('pull', 'tear', or 'strain') or contusion due to direct trauma. In both types of injury local haemorrhage is often prominent. Muscle strains are more likely to produce bleeding confined within the muscle, while external trauma often leads to more superficial, visible haematomas. The most obvious physical signs are local swelling, tenderness, pain on movement and loss of function. In the rare case of complete rupture a gap may be felt between the torn ends. The muscles most commonly involved in sports injuries are the semi-membranosus, semi-tendinosus, rectus femoris, and gastrocnemius.

Treatment consists of the relief of pain, which is often out of proportion to the degree of damage, and the R.I.C.E. measures outlined above. Surgical repair of even completely ruptured muscles gives generally disappointing results. The use of massage in order to disperse haematomas is often recommended, but its effectiveness is unproven. The same is probably true of the use of enzyme preparations such as Varidase or Chymoral. The more severe tears will need carefully graded rehabilitation under the supervision of a physiotherapist.

Bony injuries

The diagnosis and management of fractures generally is outside the scope of this chapter. All doctors should be familiar with the simple rules concerning the first-aid management of spinal injuries. Serious spinal injuries are most common at the cervical level, and some 20 per cent of these are related to sport. The on-the-spot management and methods of evacuation are well summarized by Swain, Grundy and Russell (1985a and b). When a cervical spine injury is suspected the head should be maintained in the neutral position by gentle longitudinal traction while the patient is placed supine and the airway cleared. Partial respiratory paralysis may make the use of respiratory depressant analgesics dangerous (pentazocine is probably safest). Furthermore, clearing the airway by suction can cause cardiac arrest through vagal stimulation. Four people should lift the patient: one each for the legs, hips and abdomen, shoulders, and head and neck. The last directs movements. With extensive neurological damage hypothermia and pressure damage to anaesthetic areas are other hazards. Any suspicion of cervical spine damage on the playing field demands meticulous radiology to exclude a fracture.

If there is suspicion of injury to the thoracic or lumbar spine the patient should be transported supine on a stretcher, in the anatomical position, with sandbags or other padding to prevent jolting and further injury to the cord.

Joint injuries

Sports injuries may result in a very wide variety of joint lesions, involving ligaments, bone, cartilage or haemorrhage. The most commonly damaged joints are the knee and the ankle, and the individual lesions at these sites are discussed in the chapters dealing with these regions.

The doctor attending a sportsman or woman with an injured joint has the important responsibility of deciding whether or not the injury requires transfer to hospital for investigation and/or management. At the knee and the ankle, particularly, it is wise to seek a specialist opinion if in doubt. At both these sites it is critical to differentiate between a strain and a complete rupture of a ligament. Both will produce pain when the joint is stressed in the direction which should put the ligament under tension. In theory only a complete rupture causes laxity of the movement. However, pain due to the injury, including a haemarthrosis, may make it very difficult to elicit this sign. A final decision may require examination of the joint under anaesthesia, using X-rays to confirm the degree of any laxity. X-rays may also reveal fractures or the avulsion of bone fragments at the point of insertion of ligaments. It is important to appreciate that complete ligamentous tears may result in less dramatic physical signs than partial tears.

Damage to a knee meniscus usually presents as acute pain, followed by swelling (effusion) which lasts days or weeks. Subsequent episodes of 'locking' or 'giving way' (again followed by swelling) point to the need for surgical intervention. It is useful to be familiar with the McMurray manoeuvre' (p. 189) for 'unlocking' a knee in which a fragment of torn cartilage has become trapped.

Traumatic haemarthroses, particularly if tense, can be excessively painful, and require aspiration without delay. This can be done by the doctor if he has the necessary equipment with him. However, the presence of a bleed of this magnitude into a joint is itself an indication of the possibility of serious structural damage and the need for X-ray examination.

REFERENCES

Astrand, P. O. and Rodahl, K. (1977). *Textbook of Work Physiology.* (2nd edn). McGraw-Hill, New York.

Drugs and Therapeut. Bull. (1983). More on muscle cramps. **21**, 83–4.

Swain, A., Grundy, D., and Russell, J. (1985a). ABC of spinal cord injuries: At the accident. *Br. med. J.* **291**, 1558–60.

Swain, A., Grundy, D., and Russell, J. (1985b). ABC of spinal cord injuries: Evacuation and initial management at hospital. *Br. med. J.* **291**, 1623–5.

Williams, J. G. P. and Sperryn, P. N. (eds) (1976). *Sports Medicine.* (2nd edn). Edward Arnold, London.

17 Management and referral

This chapter considers the effects of a chronic rheumatic complaint on a person's life, and how GPs and others in primary health care can help to mitigate them. It deals in turn with: social and psychological adjustment to chronic disease; specific forms of medical management; and referral to other agencies.

Disability and handicap

The pathological process of a rheumatic disease commonly brings a loss or reduction in functional ability (such as a limp or a weak grip). This is a *disability. Handicap* is the wider range of disadvantage and restriction of activity which may be brought on by disability.

A disability commonly leads to a number of disadvantages which together produce a handicap. It is in this sense that the disease impinges on the psychological and social dimension of a persons life. These aspects of a condition are often the ones that are particularly hard to assess and influence. A patient may be only mildly disabled, but will become badly handicapped if the disease and the patient's response to it brings serious disorder in the social and psychological sphere (Fig. 17.1).

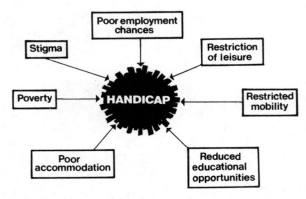

Fig. 17.1. The effects of disability. The circle of deprivation and reduced life chances.

214

Adjustment to chronic disease

The response of an individual to the effects of chronic disease can be infinitely variable, and the temptation to categorize patients' responses prematurely should be vigorously resisted. However, it is helpful to identify some response patterns which may need to be either supported or challenged.

The emotional response may be one of depression. Loss of health and the ability to do things sometimes brings on a response similar to that seen in a bereaved person. In the first stage of this response there may be numbness interspersed with anger. This is followed by a state of 'painful pining', which includes depression, self-reproach, and sometimes a search for a scapegoat. The final stage involves a process of adaptation to altered circumstances. This model can be helpful in making sense of some of the emotions the patient may go through during the first year of a chronic illness. Alternatively, the patient may develop phobic anxiety about his condition: he may be continually aware of small somatic changes and become hypochondriacal about their significance, or he may avoid many situations for fear of bringing on symptoms.

The cognitive response is also important (In what ways does the patient think about his condition? How does he cope with the worry of it? Does he use denial, projection or other defence mechanisms? Does his idea of illness prevent him from making good use of the services available?) as is the response to the disease of family members and others involved. If a patient can only get the attention he wants when his condition is bad, there will be obvious gains from maintaining disability. It is not uncommon for families and the medical profession to provide social reinforcement for the maintenance of disability.

A case history will illustrate that medical management and social intervention need to work in combination if handicap is to be successfully managed:

Mrs D was a 69-year-old widow. Osteoarthritis affected her right hip and both knees. She lived alone in a first floor council flat without lifts. She had no local family, but saw friends regularly at a local lunch club. Her GP was asked to call because she had not been out of the house for several weeks and was said to be neglecting herself. The GP discovered that she had stayed in because walking was too painful due to the combination of her osteoarthritis with painful interdigital corns and an inflamed bunion. She was seen urgently by the chiropodist, and the community physiotherapists gave her a walking stick and mobility education. However, she had lost her confidence about going out and thought she would be mugged because she walked so slowly.

A request was made for transfer to a ground floor flat and, meanwhile, efforts were made to get a lift installed in the block. She agreed to consider surgery and was put on a waiting list for a total hip replacement. Over the next year, whilst waiting for surgery and a housing transfer, she only ventured out two or three times. She had meals-on-wheels, a home help and a regular bathing aide, but became depressed and hypochondriacal about her condition. She made a good physical recovery from surgery eighteen months later but still lacked the confidence to manage the stairs to her flat. She became angry and miserable, feeling she had been through surgery but was still housebound. Not until two years after surgery was she offered a housing transfer, slightly out of her area. She took it, but found it was too far to walk to her club. A few months later she died of a myocardial infarct.

Provision

Much statutory provision exists to minimize the handicaps of the disabled person. The GP needs to know something of what is available and should be able to advise the patient where best to go for further local advice.

Social security benefits

Apart from sickness benefit and the invalidity benefit which replaces it after twenty-eight weeks, a number of non-contributory benefits are available. These include supplementary benefit, mobility allowance, and attendance allowance. A minority of the disabled are also able to claim for industrial-injuries benefit.

Employment

The disabled person is at a disadvantage in the job market and is particularly vulnerable at a time of high unemployment. The Disablement Resettlement Officer is able to recommend placement at an Employment Rehabilitation Centre, or place a client in 'sheltered work'. There is also a requirement for business of a certain size to keep a quota of their jobs for the disabled.

Accommodation

Only a minority of the disabled live in purpose-built housing. Every GP is aware of the problems caused by inappropriate housing and the difficulty of negotiating changes. Housing Authorities, on their limited budgets, are responsible for structural alterations and adaptations, whereas the Social Services Departments are responsible for aids. Assessment by the community occupational therapist helps ensure the best choice of aids, and they will also give the patient help and advice in using them appropriately.

Leisure

Restricted mobility can limit the pleasurable use of leisure time. Problems may range from the difficulty of handling small objects such as cutlery, door knobs, and normal toilets, to the restrictions of travel imposed by a patient confined to a wheelchair. What these examples demonstrate is the diminished reserves a disabled person has: a small change in mobility may cause disproportionate alterations in lifestyle. A considerable range of voluntary and other organizations, including local authorities, now provide holidays and home-based leisure activities for the disabled.

MEDICAL MANAGEMENT

Careful attention to diagnosis is central to effective medical management. However, the diagnosis should not be confined to the physical condition: it should include comment on the psychological and social factors which also need attention and possibly intervention. Close attention to what the patient says will often indicate where help is needed. As discussed in Chapter 1, special attention needs to be paid to the patient's view of his illness and what expectations he has of the medical profession if an effective therapeutic alliance is to be achieved.

For some rheumatic conditions specific therapy is indicated (e.g. allpurinol for gout, steroids for temporal arteritis), but for many conditions specific curative treatment is not available. Physicians have then to adjust their management aims towards support and prevention rather than cure.

Aims might include:

Relief of pain.
Prevention of complications and further disability.
Minimizing the degree of handicap caused by the patient's disabilities.
Helping the patient to take appropriate responsibility for his condition.
Helping and advising on the adjustment of the patient and family to chronic disease.

Pain, and the limitation of mobility which pain brings, are the two commonest presenting symptoms of rheumatic disease. The assessment and alleviation of pain is one of the primary tasks of the clinician. This can be very difficult: pain is a subjective experience and the physician can only hear verbal descriptions and see behavioural expressions. It is difficult enough for anyone to remember exactly how bad their pain was week-by-week. In addition there are cultural differences in the expression of pain, and the amount of pain that a given condition causes can be enormously variable depending on the patient's mood, personality, and the stresses which may be occurring in her life at that time. If the clinician is to assess changes in the pain then he must have some form of measurement. Two methods will be mentioned here.

The pain scale (Fig. 17.2)

This is an expression of the patient's subjective sensation of pain. The patient is asked to indicate on a linear scale how much pain he has now (either in a particular joint or the whole body). This method is a fairly reliable means of looking at changes in an individual's pain over a period of time.

Place a mark on the line to indicate how much pain you have.

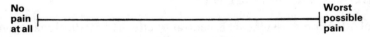

Fig. 17.2. A visual analogue pain scale.

Functional assessment

This looks at the disability that pain brings. A brief questionnaire including questions about the patient's ability to wash, dress, cook, and get about can be used. Or more simply the patient can be asked to think of something she can now do (or is unable to do) since the last visit (see Appendix 2 for further details).

The management of pain involves considering a wide range of approaches, which include:

(a) Drugs.
(b) Physical treatment.
(c) Surgery.
(d) Environmental and social modification.
(e) Psychological adjustment.

Environmental modification and psychological adjustment have been considered above. Surgery often gives enormous relief from pain; the details of the large number of procedures available are outside the scope of this book. Indications for specific operations have been mentioned in the chapters on specific conditions. A good review can be found in Freeman (1986).

DRUG TREATMENT

Analgesic and anti-inflammatory drugs

For most of the self-limiting soft tissue injuries, and for many patients with osteoarthritis, simple analgesics such as paracetamol or aspirin are suitable. Many patients choose, in addition, to buy rubefacients, analgesic sprays or heat pads. These work on the physiological principle of counter-irritation. Whether pain is deep seated or superficial it is relieved by anything which produces irritation of the skin (see p. 226). These physical methods of producing analgesia should be fully explained as their usefulness is often underestimated, and patients may inappropriately seek strong drugs instead. Patients should be encouraged to buy something cheap (such as 'white linament') or use hot water bottles, ice packs, hot baths, electric heat pads, and scarves. Many of the techniques used by physiotherapists rely on the same physiological principle. Patients should be clear that these are temporary pain-relieving mechanisms and not cures.

The non-steroidal anti-inflammatory drugs have both analgesic and anti-inflammatory properties. Taken as a single dose they have analgesic power comparable to paracetamol. Taken on a regular basis they also have an anti-inflammatory effect. The full anti-inflammatory effect is not achieved until the patients have had seven to ten days of continuous medication and failure to obtain full benefit is sometimes due to patients taking the drugs 'on demand' rather than on a regular basis. The differences in potency of anti-inflammatory effect between the various compounds are not large (although clinical efficacy correlates with the incidence of side-effects). They all have a similar potency to aspirin when taken in anti-inflammatory doses (four or more grams a day). There is, however, considerable variation in patient response, so it is well worth trying a range to find one that suits a particular patient.

Historically, high-dose aspirin was the initial treatment of choice for acute or chronic rheumatic conditions. Nowadays most doctors will start with non-steroidal anti-inflammatory drugs as they are better tolerated, and are safer in overdose. More than 50 per cent of people will have side-effects from high-dose aspirin, compared to about 30 per cent of patients on non-steroidal anti-inflammatory drugs. It is important to become well acquainted with a handful of these drugs. An expanding number of very similar products are now on the market and their benefits over the established drugs is not proven. Some of them prove to have serious side-effects—benoxaprofen (Opren) is a good example: after passing the clinical tests required by current legislation in 1980, Opren was suspended after only eighteen months of clinical use. Cutaneous side-effects were seen in 60 to 70 per cent of patients, and a number of deaths among the elderly were caused by hepatocellular damage.

Table 17.1 lists the commoner drugs with their recommended dosages. Phenylbutazone, and its related compounds, have been omitted. This drug was a first generation non-steroidal anti-inflammatory. It has a high incidence of side-effects including aplastic anaemia. Now that so many alternatives are available, there is no indication for it to be prescribed in general practice.

Table 17.1. *A selection of commonly used non-steroidal anti-inflammatory drugs*

NSAID	Strength	Recommended dose
Indomethacin (Indocid)	25 mg, 50 mg, 75 mg SR 100 mg suppository	Up to 200 mg daily
Ibuprofen (Brufen)	200 mg, 400 mg, 600 mg 100 mg/5 ml suspension	1.2 g to 2 g daily t.d.s. dose
Ketoprofen (Orudis)	50 mg, 100 mg 100 mg suppository	Up to 200 mg a day t.d.s. dose
Fenbufen (Lederfen)	300 mg	Up to 900 mg a day b.d. dose
Naproxen (Naprosyn)	250 mg, 500 mg 500 mg suppository 125 mg/5 ml suspension	Up to 1 g a day b.d. or t.d.s.
Piroxicam (Feldene)	10 mg, 20 mg 20 mg suppository	20–30 mg a day single or b.d. dose
Diclofenac (Voltarol)	25 mg, 50 mg, 100 mg SR 100 mg suppository	Up to 150 mg a day b.d. or t.d.s.

Side-effects

The anti-inflammatory action of the non-steroidal anti-inflammatory drugs is due to the inhibition of prostaglandin synthesis and other mediators of inflammation. The common side-effects of these drugs stem from their anti-prostaglandin activity, and are shared by all members of the class. Those with the greatest anti-inflammatory activity have the highest frequency of side-effects. They are listed here in order of frequency.

1. Gastric irritation, erosion and ulceration. For indomethacin, rates of gastric intolerance may be as high as 30 per cent, for ibuprofen which is less potent, around 15 per cent.
2. CNS effects, headaches, dizziness, muzziness. These are thought to be due to cerebral salt and water retention.
3. Hypersensitivity reactions. Rashes, asthma, rhinitis.
4. Renal. Anti-prostaglandin activity causes decreased renal perfusion and salt and water retention. This may precipitate oedema or cardiac failure, particularly in the elderly. A slight rise in blood urea is almost invariable.

Systemic steroids

Steroids are by far the most powerful suppressors of inflammation, and also have an immunosuppressive effect. Although they may give excellent symptomatic relief in many chronic rheumatic conditions, they should only be used where there are specific indications. Not only are there well known and serious side-effects, but in many conditions the illness worsens as the dose is reduced. Once started it may be very difficult to reduce the dose or withdraw the drug.

Major side-effects of corticosteroids:

1. Gastro-intestinal (peptic ulceration).
2. Endocrine (Cushingoid apearance, diabetes, growth disturbance, adrenal suppression, loss of resistance to infections).
3. Mineralocorticoid (hypertension, fluid retention, potassium loss).
4. Musculoskeletal (steroid myopathy, osteoporosis leading to fractures, aseptic necrosis).
5. Neurological (euphoria, steroid psychosis).

Oral steroids are the treatment of choice in temporal arteritis and polymyalgia, in these conditions early treatment may prevent the onset of blindness. Steroids, alone or in combination with other immunosuppressive drugs, are used in the systemic connective tissue disorders, SLE, polyarteritis, polymyositis, and dermatomyositis. These conditions are rare in general practice, and initiation of these treatments should always be in consultation with a specialist. Steroids should not be used in ankylosing spondylitis, psoriatic arthropathy or the other chronic inflammatory arthropathies. Their place in the treatment of rheumatoid disease is limited. Wherever possible the dose should be kept to a minimum, not more than 7.5 mg of prednisone a day, and because of the side-effects should be restricted to the following situations:

Severe systemic effects (vasculitis, eye problems).
To prevent gross loss of function, or immobilization in a wheelchair.
In the elderly where the quality of remaining life may be most important.
When other drug treatment has failed to control intolerable pain and inflammation.

Local steroid injections

The use of local steroid injections in the surgery enables the GP to treat many of the minor but distressing conditions which otherwise get referred to rheumatology or orthopaedic outpatient departments. The benefits of local injection far outweigh the disadvantages; technique is simple and can be gained from a book. Local hospitals with an 'injection clinic' may allow the GP to gain experience under supervision. Most synovial joints can be aspirated or injected, and the infiltration of soft tissue lesions is also straightforward. (For details of technique see p. 189 for the knee and p. 154 for the shoulder joint.)

The main indications for local steroid injections are:

(a) An inflammatory polyarthritis where one or two joints are not responding to systemic treatment.
(b) Monoarthritis.
(c) Mild degenerative joint disease, especially where there is an additional acute synovitis, possibly triggered by debris in the joint.
(d) Crystal synovitis.
(e) Tendinitis. Injections should be into the tendon sheath or around the tendon but not into the tendon itself, because injections into a weakened tendon may cause rupture. This is a recognized hazard with inappropriately placed Achilles' tendon injections (p. 198).
(f) Enthesopathies, tennis elbow, golfer's elbow, plantar fasciitis. Injection of a small volume at the site of maximum pain seems most successful (p. 169).

What to use

A single dose ampule should always be used to avoid the risk of contamination. The preparations in common use include:

Hydrocortisone acetate (25 mg/ml). This has a claimed duration of 10 days. Short-acting compounds such as this are preferred for local infiltration as the powerful long-acting compounds can cause local skin atrophy.
Methyl prednisolone acetate (depo-medrone 40 mg/ml). This is said to last for about 21 days.
Triamcinolone hexacetonide (Lederspan 5 mg/ml or 20 mg/ml). This lasts up to 90 days. It is particularly suitable for intra-articular injection.

It is a matter of clinical choice whether to use local anaesthetic for intra-articular injections. When infiltrating soft tissue lesions local anaesthetic can be a useful diagnostic guide as to whether the injection has been accurately placed.

Routine aseptic precautions should always be observed. Use disposable needles and syringes, and if injecting an insoluble preparation such as hydrocortisone acetate, a gauge 23 (blue) is the narrowest needle through which the preparation will pass. The skin should be cleansed with an antiseptic, and the puncture site covered with an adhesive dressing for twenty-four hours. Using these simple precautions both intra-articular and soft tissue injection has proved remarkably safe. The main hazards include:

1. Introducing infection. This is very rare but very serious. It should be suspected if the joint is inflamed and much more painful following an injection. This may be confused with a 'crystal synovitis' reaction which occasionally follows the injection of corticosteroids. Aspiration for microscopy will be diagnostic.
2. There is evidence that very frequent injections may cause damage in some joints. Aseptic necrosis of the femoral head has been recorded, and a Charcot-type of arthropathy in weight-bearing joints. However, if injections are performed as often as four times a year there is little evidence that damage is caused.

Remission inducing drugs used in rheumatoid arthritis

Gold

Sodium aurothiomalate injections work over a period of months and are thought to modify and retard the disease process. How gold works is unknown. The response is unpredictable for any individual, but if there is no response within three months it is not worth continuing. Following weekly test doses of 10 mg and 20 mg, the patient is given 50 mg weekly by deep intramuscular injection until a total dose of 500 mg is reached. The injections can then be reduced in frequency, (e.g. to 50 mg a month), depending on the response. Gold should be continued as long as there is a response, it is no longer customary to think of a finite course of injections.

An initial remission can be expected in 60 per cent of patients, but side-effects occur in about 25 per cent. Complete recovery from these is usual, with adequate monitoring, and serious consequences are rare. The commonest side-effects are:

1. Rashes. These are often heralded by pruritis and eosinophilia, and include urticaria, vesicular or eczematous erruptions, buccal ulceration, and, occasionally, exfoliative dermatitis.
2. Proteinuria. This occurs in about 5–10 per cent of patients and is usually reversible on stopping the injections. Only rarely does it progress to a nephrotic syndrome.
3. Thrombocytopenia and, rarely, progressive suppression of the bone marrow.

Every patient having gold injections should carry a gold card (c.f. steroid cards). Before every injection the doctor should enquire about rashes, and test the urine for protein (patients can be prescribed Albustix and asked to test their urine weekly, a trace of albumen should be ignored). A full blood count including platelets should be done monthly during regular injections. The injections should be stopped if the platelet count drops below $0.15 \times 10^9/l$ (check normal range with local laboratory).

Cautious re-introduction can be attempted if the count rapidly returns to normal.

Penicillamine

The mode of action of this drug remains obscure, but as an oral preparation it has advantages over gold injections for some patients. The usual dose regimen is to start with 125 mg o.d. and, with monthly increments of 125 mg, to work up to 500 mg. As with gold, partial remission can be expected in 60 per cent, but there are side-effects in about one third of patients. Loss of taste can be particularly distressing although it usually settles if treatment is continued. Rashes, proteinuria, and marrow suppression are the serious side-effects, and a regular routine of testing the urine and blood count should be adhered to.

Less commonly used drugs

Chloroquine

Used for rheumatoid arthritis in some centres. It is a weaker but safer drug than gold or penicillamine. Regular ophthalmic checks are mandatory to monitor for retinal damage due to dose-related pigment deposition on the choroid.

Azathioprine, chlorambucil, and cyclophosphamide

These drugs are used in severe, resistant cases of rheumatoid disease, and as immunosuppressants in other connective tissue disorders. The main hazards of these cytotoxic drugs are marrow suppression and the risk of inducing malignancy.

Sulphasalazine

This is now being tested as a potentially useful remission-inducing drug. Given as enteric-coated 500 mg tablets, the starting dose is 500 mg daily, increasing in weekly steps to about 1 g t.d.s. Three-monthly blood counts and liver function tests are advisable.

PHYSICAL METHODS OF TREATMENT

Under this heading will be considered the role of the physiotherapist and a number of physical therapies, such as manipulation and acupuncture, which have traditionally been seen as fringe treatments outside the NHS. In the last few decades the emphasis has shifted away from physical methods of treating chronic rheumatic complaints towards medical and drug treatment. This reflects increased knowledge of the pathological processes associated with rheumatic diseases, and the expectation that abnormalities can be reversed by specific pharmacological manipulation.

There is now a move back to the use of physical methods, with considerable public interest in 'alternative' therapies. Some of these are now coming under scrutiny in controlled trials, but until the indications for them and their efficacy are known, informed scepticism is probably the most appropriate stance.

Physiotherapy

Physiotherapy is the use of physical methods to produce improvement in function of the locomotor system. Unlike many of the 'alternative' therapies, its philosophy has remained within the orthodox, empirical, medical model. Physiotherapists have worked alongside the medical profession since the end of the nineteenth century.

The role of physiotherapists has changed considerably in recent years. First, many departments now take referrals directly from GPs. In most health districts this has been successful, and referrals have been appropriate. The second important change is that physiotherapists are deciding for themselves what form of physical treatment to use on a patient, and no longer simply providing a treatment regimen prescribed by the doctor. This new independence should allow the profession to incorporate the most useful methods from the 'fringe' into orthodox treatment programmes.

Physiotherapy can be divided into three aspects:

Educational

The special skills of physiotherapists are clearly seen here. Advice on how to do things is of more value than doing them for the patient. For example, for a patient with low back pain, a 'back life class' which gives advice on getting out of bed, posture, lifting, and exercises to do at home, may be more beneficial in prevention than brief treatment sessions in an Outpatient Department which ease the symptoms for a short while only. Other areas where prevention by education is important are: teaching patients with rheumatoid disease how to use their hands without damaging the joints; advice on mobility aids and their proper use; and relaxation techniques for any patient with painful joints and tense muscles.

Specific treatments

Physiotherapists have an essential role in the instruction and supervision of patients with joint disease whose muscles have become weakened by pain and disuse. Active, resisted exercises build up muscle bulk which improves joint stability and often reduces pain. Various techniques for heating the tissues may also be used, such as ultrasound, short-wave diathermy, wax baths and hydrotherapy. Whether or not some of these techniques have a specific effect is as yet uncertain. What is certain is that these methods suppress pain in the short-term and so are an important adjunct to improving mobility and exercise tolerance, which, in turn, improve motivation.

Psychosocial treatment

The physiotherapist has time to give, and during physical treatments is able to lay hands on the patient. For centuries these elements of therapy have been recognized as central to the process of healing. Many physiotherapists have, in addition, gained considerable knowledge of counselling skills. These aspects of physiotherapy can be put to use in helping the patient adapt to the process of increasing disability and all the painful emotions this engenders. They can also be harnessed in helping the patient with chronic pain. Sympathetic attention to the patient will often enable the physiotherapist to encourage the use of simple pain relieving techniques, or advise on acceptable changes in lifestyle, and to help in the appropriate administration of drug therapy.

ALTERNATIVE THERAPIES

As some 30 per cent of patients with chronic rheumatic diseases will consult an alternative practitioner, it is important for GPs to know about the commoner forms of therapy. Many patients will ask their GP's opinion before going ahead, and some GPs are making informal referrals to alternative practitioners. If this is being done it is essential for the practitioner to know about the credentials of the therapist and to have an informed opinion of the efficacy of the treatment offered.

Acupuncture

Considerable interest in acupuncture as a method of analgesia has meant that the technique has begun to be investigated in the West; controlled trials of its efficacy in various conditions are just beginning.

Current neurophysiological explanations for acupuncture analgesia rely on the discovery of the endorphin neurotransmittors, and the theories of pain transmission developed by Melzack and Wall. Their gate-control theory of pain, developed in the 1960s, states that pain sensation is carried in unmyelinated C fibres, and light touch in myelinated A fibres. These modalities are integrated in the dorsal horn of the spinal cord. The onward transmission of pain is controlled by the balance of activity in A and C fibres. If A fibres are stimulated by acupuncture, transcutaneous electrical nerve stimulation (TENS), or counter-irritants, then the onward transmission of pain is partially suppressed.

In addition to this peripheral system there are endorphin-mediated descending pathways which arise within the reticular activating system and the cerebral nuclei. These are capable of exerting inhibitory and analgesic effects on the activity of the dorsal horn. In the present state of knowledge it appears that acupuncture, in common with TENS (where the stimulus is applied to the skin surface rather than through needles), promotes the release of endogenous opiates within the brain. These are thought to activate the descending neuronal pathways which inhibit the activity of the pain pathways in the dorsal horn (see Leweth 1985).

Is acupuncture more than a placebo?

This question has an unexpected twist as there is now evidence that the placebo response (which gives significant pain relief to about one third of patients) is mediated by endorphin release, and can be blocked by naloxone (see Levine *et al.* 1978). Good, controlled trials of the effectiveness of acupuncture analgesia are yet to be done, even though it is already available as a treatment for chronic pain at some regional pain clinics. It is difficult to predict how an individual will respond to acupuncture: some appear to gain immediate analgesia, for others the effect starts slowly and may last a long time.

Manipulative treatment

'Manipulation' means skilful or dextrous treatment by the hand. Manipulative treatment in one form or another has been carried out since the time of the ancient Greeks. Nowadays it is performed by a variety of practitioners: physiotherapists who have a special interest in the technique, or lay manipulators such as osteopaths or chiropracters who are usually not medically qualified. Manipulative treatments can be grouped under three headings:

1. Soft tissue techniques. These include massage and friction.
2. Mobilizations. These are gentle movements, usually repetitive and oscillatory, which relax muscles and elongate tight structures (Fig. 17.3).
3. Manipulation. A single, high velocity thrust which causes rapid movement in a joint and soft tissues (Fig. 17.4).

Osteopathy

Osteopathy is a system of diagnosis and treatment in which manual treatment, along with attention to posture and exercise, are said to effect a change in the well-being of the body. Some osteopaths have wide-ranging mechanical hypotheses based on an embryological segmental

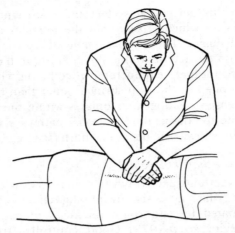

Fig. 17.3. A mobilization at the mid-lumbar level.

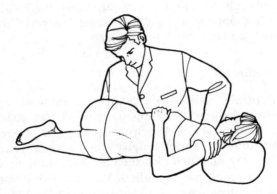

Fig. 17.4. Rotational manipulation of the lumbar spine.

analysis: thus asthma, for example, may improve with manipulation of the thoracic spine because both lie within the same body segment. Many osteopaths put less emphasis on this theoretical framework than once they did.

The benefits of osteopathy seem to come in part from the physical techniques, but also from the time and attention paid to the patient and the general advice on lifestyle. Much of the healing attributed to osteopathy (or other manual practitioners) can be considered as a form of 'manual psychotherapy'. At present anyone can call himself an osteopath, but only graduates of the British or European School of Osteopathy are entitled to the designation MRO (Member of the Register of Osteopaths).

Does osteopathy work?

This is often asked, and may be as difficult to answer as the question 'Does a general practice consultation work?'. If the manipulative techniques are isolated from other aspects of treatment there is no convincing evidence for long-term benefits. One recent trial compared the outcome of three groups of patients with low back pain when treated with short-wave diathermy, osteopathy, and non-functioning short-wave diathermy. The results showed that over 50 per cent of patients improved on all three different regimens. This result is larger than might be expected from a placebo response alone, and is probably explained by the benefit of regular patient–therapist contact. It is this aspect of osteopathy and other alternative therapies which is much more difficult to assess by conventional trials than are specific techniques.

A GP considering referral to an osteopath, either for back pain or for a stress-related condition should:

Make sure the osteopath is a Member of the Register of Osteopaths.
Get to know the techniques he uses. A wide range of manoeuvres are available, some of them rather esoteric.
Continue to assess and treat the patient him or herself.

Chiropractors

Chiropraxy has for its theoretical basis the idea that spinal subluxation can cause disease in various distant organs. Thus spinal 'adjustments' and manipulations become treatments for a wide range of diseases. Chiropracters take their own X-rays and have a special system for analysing them to pinpoint spinal abnormalities. Treatment is usually by high velocity, forceful manipulations. Many of their theories are quite incompatible with orthodox empirical medicine, and as yet there have been no controlled trials of chiropraxy.

REFERENCES

Darnborough, A. and Kinrade, D. (1979). *Directory for the disabled.* Woodhead-Faulkener for the Royal Society for Disability and Rehabilitation.
Dukes, M. N. G. (ed.) (1984). *Meyler's side-effects of drugs.*
Freeman, M. A. R. (1986). Operative surgery in the rheumatic diseases. In *Mason and Currey's Clinical Rheumatology* (4th edn) Currey H. L. F. (ed.). Churchill Livingstone, London.
Glossop, E. (1977). Prescribing physiotherapy. *Hospital Update.* **3**, 593–5.
Hasler, J. and Schofield, T. (eds) (1984). *Continuing Care: The Management of Chronic Disease.* Oxford University Press, Oxford.
Lewith, G. T. (1981). How does acupuncture work? *Br. med. J.* **283**, 746–74.

Lewith, G. T. (ed.) (1985). *Alternative Therapies*. Heinemann, London.
Levine, J., Gordon, N., *et al.* (1978). The mechanism of placebo analgesia. *Lancet*. **II**, 654–7.
Reports on rheumatic diseases (1982). Nos. 81 and 82. Arthritis and Rheumatism Council, London.
Yates, D. A. H. (1977). The use of local steroid injections. *Br. med. J.* **1**, 495–6.

Appendix 1. Investigations

HAEMATOLOGY

Erythrocyte sedimentation rate (ESR)

The ESR remains a valuable, if non-specific, screening test for inflammatory and certain other rheumatic diseases. It is also a useful means of assessing the active inflammatory component of a condition such as rheumatoid arthritis. The standard Westergren technique involves diluting blood with a citrate solution as anticoagulant, then drawing it up into a 200 mm glass tube which is left standing vertically for one hour. The distance in mm to which the upper border of the red cell column has settled is recorded as the ESR. The upper limit of normal is somewhere between 10 and 20 mm/hour. Various factors influence the rate at which the erythrocytes sediment and, as an example, the accelerated ESR in rheumatoid arthritis is due to a combination of:

Increased fibrinogen levels (an 'acute-phase reactant' response to inflammation).
Increased immunoglobulin levels (reflecting immunological activity).
Lowered numbers of red cells (reflecting, particularly, the effect of a chronic illness on the bone marrow).

Other tests have been proposed as alternatives to the ESR. Thus, some laboratories record plasma viscosity, others C-reactive protein levels (an acute-phase reactant which responds more promptly than fibrinogen levels to changes in inflammatory activity). However, for the time being the ESR is unlikely to be replaced as the most useful screening test.

In patients complaining of skeletal types of pain an elevated ESR may be the first clue to conditions such as:

Inflammatory arthropathies, e.g. rheumatoid arthritis.
Polymyalgia rheumatica.
Multiple myelomatosis (elevated levels of circulating immunoglobulins) or other disseminated malignancies.
Concealed infection.
Systemic connective tissue disorders (SLE, polyarteritis, dermatomyositis, etc.).

In patients apparently suffering from degenerative joint complaints the

231

ESR thus provides an invaluable screening test for excluding more serious underlying conditions.

The blood count

Blood counts are used in rheumatic diseases particularly for monitoring drug therapy. The white cell count may also provide useful diagnostic pointers such as leucopenia in SLE and Felty's syndrome, and leucocytosis or eosinophilia in polyarteritis nodosa.

Many inflammatory rheumatic diseases are associated with anaemia, but interpretation of low haemoglobin levels in conditions such as rheumatoid arthritis can be difficult. True iron deficiency may result from drug-induced gastrointestinal blood loss, or the sick bone marrow may be unable to use the available iron stores. In both instances the peripheral blood smear may appear hypochromic and microcytic, so reliance cannot be placed on this. The 'gold standard' for true iron deficiency is the presence or absence of stainable iron in the bone marrow. However, two less invasive tests can provide this information indirectly: anaemic rheumatoid patients are likely to respond to iron therapy if they have (1) a total iron-binding capacity (TIBC) greater than 55 µmol/l and (2) a serum ferritin level of less than 55 µg/l.

IMMUNOLOGICAL TESTS

Rheumatoid factors

These are autoantibodies directed against immunoglobulin G (IgG), which can be detected in the serum of about 85 per cent of patients with rheumatoid arthritis. In the standard laboratory tests IgG is attached to a marker (sheep erythrocytes in the 'sheep cell' tests and polystyrene particles in the 'Latex' test). Agglutination titres of $\geq 1/16$ are significant in the sheep cell tests, $\geq 1/80$ in the Latex test. These tests reveal the presence of rheumatoid factors in the IgM class only. Using other techniques they can be shown to be present in the other immunoglobulin classes. Positive tests (usually in low titres) may occur in other autoimmune diseases, in liver disease (viral hepatitis, cirrhosis, chronic active hepatitis), or occasionally in healthy subjects (5 per cent).

These tests tend to become positive early in the course of rheumatoid arthritis, and then remain positive (unless reversed by drugs such as penicillamine). They are often present in high titre and provide both an invaluable aid to diagnosis, and a pointer to prognosis (those with higher titres tend to fare worse).

Antibodies to nuclear antigens

The sera of patients suffering from SLE usually contain a variety of auto-antibodies. The most characteristic are those directed against some component of the cell nucleus. There are three standard tests for these antibodies:

The LE-cell test

Peripheral blood leucocytes are incubated, then smeared, stained, and examined for the presence of polymorphs which have phagocytosed (and become distended by) nuclear material from disrupted cells. This phenomenon depends on the opsonization of the nuclear material by anti-nuclear antibodies. This remains a valid test for SLE, but it is very demanding on laboratory staff time and for that reason is seldom used.

The fluorescent anti-nuclear antibody test (ANA, ANF)

In this two-stage test the first step involves exposing a frozen section of animal tissue (e.g. rat kidney) to different dilutions of the patient's serum; any anti-nuclear antibody fixes to the cell nuclei in the section. In the second stage the section, after washing, is exposed to a fluoroscein-linked goat anti-human immunoglobulin antiserum. This will attach to any human immunoglobulin fixed to the section. The section is then examined by ultraviolet light microscopy. Bright green fluoresence of the cell nuclei marks where antibody is attached and hence indicates a positive test. Results are expressed either as titres (1/40 being positive), or in international units (25 iu being positive). A 'speckled' pattern of nuclear staining is suggestive of an antibody to an 'extractable nuclear antigen' (see below), and in high titre this may be a pointer to mixed connective tissue disease.

This test is highly sensitive but not very specific. Almost every active case of SLE will give a positive test, but positive results may be obtained in other connective tissue and autoimmune diseases too. It is simple, rapid and cheap to perform, and thus provides the ideal screening test for SLE. A positive result is an indication for carrying out the following test.

DNA-binding test

This is a test for the presence of autoantibodies directed specifically against native (double-stranded) DNA. The test serum is mixed with isotopically labelled bacterial dsDNA. The percentage of radioactivity 'bound' into immune complexes can then be measured and represents the DNA-binding capacity of the serum. The upper limit of normal varies between laboratories, being about 25 per cent. Levels above this are highly specific for SLE, and the higher they are, the more active the disease. The test is not very sensitive, and mild cases of SLE may give negative results. In monitoring the progress of a patient with SLE, rising levels of DNA-binding combined with falling levels of serum complement (see below) are indicators of immune-complex formation and may herald renal involvement.

Other autoantibodies

Extractable nuclear antibodies (ENA)

This term refers to a group of autoantibodies which may be found in the serum of patients suffering from autoimmune diseases. Some of the more important nuclear and cytoplasmic autoantibodies are:

Antigen	Disease associations
Sm	SLE
Ro (SSA)	SLE; Sjøgren's syndrome
La (SSB)	SLE; Sjøgren's syndrome
Nuclear ribonucleoprotein (nRNP)	Mixed connective tissue disease
Scl-70	Systemic sclerosis
Centromere	Systemic sclerosis (CREST)
Jo-1	Polymyositis

Anti-phospholipid antibodies

This is a group of autoantibodies which has recently attracted considerable attention. Two of these have been known for some time: the anti-cardiolipin antibody active in the Wassermann reaction for syphilis, and the 'lupus anticoagulant' detected in some cases of SLE. Recently developed, sensitive tests for antibodies to phospholipid have shown that these occur in patients both with and without SLE, and their presence is associated with recurrent abortions, venous and arterial thrombosis, and thrombocytopenia.

Serum complement and immune complexes

When antibodies combine with antigens to form immune complexes they may 'fix' complement and thus activate the sequence of reactions in the 'complement cascade'. This process lowers the serum levels of complement components. Low levels of serum complement are therefore an index of the formation of immune complexes in the circulation. Total haemolytic complement activity (CH_{50}), C_3 and C_4 are the measurements most commonly used.

A wide variety of tests is available to indicate the actual presence of immune complexes in the circulation. An example is the C_1q-binding test.

BIOCHEMICAL TESTS

Serum alkaline phosphatase

Elevated concentrations of alkaline phosphatase may result from abnormalities of either bone or liver. Bone alkaline phosphatase reflects osteoblastic activity (new bone formation) and elevated concentrations occur in ostemalacia, Paget's disease, hyperparathyroid bone disease, and healing fractures. In patients with skeletal pains the serum alkaline phosphatase concentration thus provides a convenient screening test for metabolic bone disease. It is, however, important to remember that it is not raised in osteoporosis (unless a bone fracture is also present). The upper limit of normal is about 100 iu in adults, but is higher in growing children.

Serum acid phosphatase

This provides a valuable screening test for the presence of bone metastases from prostatic carcinoma. The upper limit of normal for the prostatic component of acid phosphatase is 7.2 iu.

Creatine phosphokinase (CPK, CK)

CPK is released from damaged muscles and may be detected in the serum in increased quantities following a myocardial infarction, and in patients with polymyositis. It is a valuable screening test in patients suspected of having polymyositis. The upper limit of normal is about 100 iu, depending on the method.

Plasma uric acid

The upper limit of normal for uric acid in the plasma is about 420 μmol/l in men and 380 μmol/l in women. Although elevated concentrations are the underlying biochemical defect in gout, and it is uncommon for untreated cases of gout to have normal concentrations, the converse is not true. Routine biochemical screening of sera frequently gives elevated concentrations of uric acid, but most of these patients do not have gout. The diagnosis of gout should ideally be based on the identification of uric acid crystals (see below). Without identification, it requires a characteristic clinical picture in conjunction with an elevated plasma uric acid concentration to justify this diagnosis.

SYNOVIAL FLUID EXAMINATION

The diagnostic information which can be gleaned from examination of the synovial fluid is limited. It can provide a reliable diagnosis of infective arthritis or of crystal synovitis, and it may provide a pointer to whether the underlying condition is more or less inflammatory. Occasionally it may reveal an unsuspected haemarthrosis.

Gross appearance

Normal synovial fluid is clear, straw coloured, viscous, and does not clot on standing. Inflammatory synovitis produces a larger volume of fluid which is cloudy owing to the cellular content, less viscous, and which clots on standing due to the increased fibrinogen content. Blood-staining may indicate trauma, a bleeding tendency, villonodular synovitis, or (uncommonly) very acute crystal synovitis. Established septic arthritis typically yields a turbid fluid, but reliance cannot be replaced on this. The fluid may be only slightly cloudy in early cases, while uncomplicated rheumatoid or gouty fluids may sometimes appear purulent.

Protein content

The rapid appearance of a firm clot points to a high protein content. In degenerative joint disease the protein content is usually about 20–30 g/l, in inflammatory arthritis about 40–70 g/l.

Leucocytes

Synovial fluids for cell counts must immediately be well mixed with EDTA anticoagulant. There is great variation in cell counts and wide overlap between different conditions. Very roughly, in degenerative joint disease cell counts tend to be below 1×10^9/l, while in inflammatory conditions the counts are usually greater than 3×10^9/l. The proportion of neutrophils tends to be below 50 per cent in osteoarthritis, above 50 per cent in rheumatoid arthritis, and over 95 per cent in septic arthritis, but again there is wide variation.

Crystals

Fluid for crystal examination should be placed in a sterile container without anticoagulant. A good quality polarizing microscope is necessary for the examination and, if this facility is not available locally, the specimen should be mailed to a laboratory where it can be examined.

Polarizing light microscopy allows birefringent crystals to be identified and the two important types (urate and pyrophosphate) to be differentiated.

Microbiology

Synovial fluids are examined by standard microbiological techniques. When septic arthritis is suspected, both synovial fluid and blood should be obtained for culture before starting antibiotic treatment.

Tuberculous fluids often do not yield tubercle bacilli. Therefore, when tuberculosis is suspected synovial biopsy is often undertaken.

SYNOVIAL BIOPSY

Histological appearances do not differentiate between the various types of 'inflammatory' arthropathy. For this reason synovial biopsy is undertaken, mainly in cases of unexplained monarticular arthritis, in order to exclude tuberculosis. Specimens may be obtained by 'blind' needle biopsy, during arthroscopy (see below), or by open arthrotomy.

ARTHROSCOPY

Endoscopy of the knee joint allows a very complete examination of the synovium, menisci, and joint cartilage. Its main use is in the investigation of cases of internal derangement in this joint: meniscal tears, cruciate ligament lesions, and loose bodies can be readily identified.

RADIO-ISOTOPE SCANNING

Radio-isotope scanning following intravenous injection of radioactive bone-seeking material allows sites of increased bone turnover to be identified. These 'hot spots' are non-specific and do not indicate the nature of the bone lesion. The technique is particularly valuable in patients with unexplained skeletal pains in whom X-rays are negative. Both neoplastic and infective bony lesions show as 'hot spots'; so also do joints which are the sites of any type of arthropathy.

ARTHROGRAPHY

X-rays taken following injection of radio-opaque material into a joint provide a positive image of the synovial cavity. This is of value in the diagnosis of a ruptured joint cavity: in the knee the dye can be seen to track down into the calf. Better detail is obtained when a 'double-contrast' injection of dye and gas is undertaken. This can reveal a tear in a meniscus.

REFERENCES

Currey, H. L. F. and Vernon-Roberts, B. (1976). Examination of synovial fluid. *Clinics in Rheumatic Diseases.* **2**, 149–77.

Fawthrop, F., Hornby, J., Swan, A., Hutton, C. *et al.* (1985). A comparison of normal and pathological synovial fluid. *Br. J. Rheumatol.* **24**, 61–9.

Forrester, D. M. and Brown, J. C. (eds) (1983). Radiological investigations in rheumatology. *Clinics in Rheumatic Diseases* **9**, 289–483.

Garvie, M. W., Reynolds, C. P., and Turner, M. J. (1984). Advances in imaging techniques in rheumatology. *Reports on Rheumatic Diseases (No. 89)* Arthritis and Rheumatism Council, London.

Hughes, G. R. V. (1984). Autoantibodies in lupus and its variants: experience in 1000 patients. *Br. med. J.* **289**, 339–42.

Powell, R. J. (1984). Serum complement levels. *Br. J. Hosp. Med.* **32**, 104–10.

Appendix 2. Assessment of disease activity in rheumatoid arthritis

A reliable method of assessing the disease process and patient outcome in rheumatoid arthritis is badly needed. This is essential for monitoring the disease and for making decisions about changes in treatment. At present it is not known for certain which disease parameters point to a particularly good or bad prognosis. The commonly used criteria for assessing the disease in a rheumatoid patient include the following:

Clinical features. Duration of early morning stiffness; amount of pain; the number of inflamed joints; whether or not the patient thinks she has improved; grip strength; drug usage.

Laboratory tests. ESR; rheumatoid factor titre; haemoglobin; count of erosions seen on hand X-rays.

Functional ability. What the patient can and cannot do. This may be based on observation, a questionnaire, or a formal assessment by the occupational therapist.

Current research in clinical judgement analysis suggests that most clinicians pick out two or three features with which to make their clinical judgements. The question is which ones are the most reliable? At present the evidence suggests that the ESR and a simple count of the swollen and painful joints gives a good measure of disease activity at any one time.

The functional ability of a patient is not a parameter frequently assessed by clinicians in their day to day practice. However, this may be the dimension of disease with the most importance for patients. Disability can be conveniently assessed by a questionnaire such as the modified Stanford Health Assessment Questionnaire (Table 1). This has been extensively validated on patients both in the USA and in the UK, and has proved to be a sensitive way to monitor the progress of the disease and its modification by treatment. It forms a useful record of a patient's current disability and could be used at six-monthly intervals to demonstrate whether or not a slow-acting drug is of benefit to a patient.

Scoring and use of the Health Assessement Questionnaire

Most patients can fill out this questionnaire on their own.

239

Table 1. *The modified Stanford Health Assessment Questionnaire*

Please tick the one response which best describes your usual abilities over the past week

	Without any difficulty	With some difficulty	With much difficulty	Unable to do
1. DRESSING and GROOMING				
Are you able to:				
Dress yourself including shoelaces and buttons?	......	..X..	......	......
Shampoo your hair?	..X..	......	......	......
2. RISING				
Are you able to:				
Stand up from an armless straight chair?	......	......	..X..	......
Get in and out of bed?	......	......	..X..	......
3. EATING				
Are you able to:				
Cut your meat?	..X..	......	......	......
Lift a full glass to your mouth?	..X..	......	......	......
Open a new carton of milk (or soap powder)?	..X..	......	......	......
4. WALKING				
Are you able to:				
Walk outdoors on flat ground?	......	......	..X..	......
Climb up five steps?	......	......	......	..X..

Please tick any aids which you regularly use for any of these activities

Stick	..X..	Dressing aids	......
Walking frame	......	Special untensils	......
Crutches	......	Other (specify)	......
Wheelchair	......		

Please tick any categories for which you usually need help from another person

Dressing and grooming	......	Eating	......
Rising	......	Walking	......

Table 1. *Continued*

Please tick the one response which best describes your usual abilities over the past week

	Without any difficulty	With some difficulty	With much difficulty	Unable to do
5. HYGIENE				
Are you able to:				
Wash and dry your entire body?	......	..X..	......	......
Have a bath?	......	......	..X..	......
Get on and off the toilet?	......	..X..	......	......
6. REACH				
Are you able to:				
Reach and get down a 5 lb object from just above your head?	..X..	......	......	......
Bend and pick up clothes from the floor?	......	..X..	......	......
7. GRIP				
Are you able to:				
Open car doors?	..X..	......	......	......
Open jars which have previously been opened?	..X..	......	......	......
Turn taps on and off?	..X..	......	......	......
8. ACTIVITIES				
Are you able to:				
Do errands and shop?	......	......	..X..	......
Get in and out of a car?	......	......	..X..	......
Do vacuuming, housework and gardening?	......	......	..X..	......

Please tick any aids that you regularly use for any of these activities

Raised toilet seat	......	Bath rail	......
Bath seat	......	Long-handled appliances for reach	
Jar opener	......		......
Other (specify)	......	reach	

Please tick any categories for which you usually need help from another person

Hygiene	......	Gripping and opening things	......
Reach	......	Errands and Housework	..X..

The *disability index* is derived from the scores in each of the eight categories on the questionnaire. Each category has at least two component questions, each of which is marked 0 to 3 as follows:

Without any difficulty	=0
With some difficulty	=1
With much difficulty	=2
Unable to do	=3

The score for any category is the highest score obtained from any of the component questions.

If an aid or device is used for any category the score for that category is raised to 2. If help from another person is needed for any category the score for that category is raised to 3.

The disability index is calculated by adding the scores for each of the eight categories and then dividing by 8, the result will be a number between 0.0 and 3.0.

The score for the example on the questionnaire (a patient with severe hip disease) is calculated as follows:

Category	Score	
1.	1	
2.	2	
3.	0	
4.	3	
5.	2	
6.	1	
7.	0	
8.	3	(raised from 2 to 3 as help needed from
	12	another person)

Disability index (12 divided by 8) is 1.5

This example demonstrates that one can separate out upper- and lower-limb deformity, and that one can use it with a patient to identify problems for which there may be an obvious solution.

ASSESSMENT OF JOINT TENDERNESS

The number of inflamed joints in a patient with arthritis is one of the criteria used by clinicians both in clinical practice, and in clinical trials to assess response to treatment. The best known articular index is the Ritchie index devised in 1968. An example of its use is shown in Table 2.

Table 2. *Example of scoring the Ritchie articular index*

Joint		Not tender (0)	Tender (+1)	Tender and winced (+2)	Tender winced, withdrew (+3)	Joint score
Cervical spine		+				0
Temperomandibular joints			+			1
Acromioclavicular		+				0
Shoulders	(L)			+		2
	(R)			+		2
Elbows	(L)				+	3
	(R)	+				0
Wrists	(L)	+				0
	(R)			+		2
Metacarpo-phalangeal	(L)		+			1
	(R)		+			1
Phalangointer-phalangeal	(L)			+		2
	(R)			+		2
Hips	(L)	+				0
	(R)	+				0
Knees	(L)	+				0
	(R)		+			1
Ankles	(L)	+				0
	(R)		+			1
Talocalcaneal	(L)	+				0
	(R)		+			1
Mid-tarsal	(L)	+				0
	(R)				+	3
Metatarso-phalangeal	(L)		+			1
	(R)				+	3
					Total	+26

This index requires examination of the whole patient and takes at least two-and-a-half minutes to perform in practised hands. The intra-observer error rate is low, but the inter-observer error rate is high, so it is best used for repeated assessment by the same person. A recent comparison of the various indices in clinical use suggests that a simple count of the joints which are both swollen, and tender (metacarpophalangeal and metatarsophalangeal joints counted separately) gives a good enough guide to the general level of inflammation.

REFERENCES

Kirwan, J. R., Reeback, J. S. (1986). Stanford health assessment questionnaire modified to assess disability in British patients with rheumatoid arthritis. *Br. J. Rheumatol.* **25**, 206–9.

Kirwan, J. R., Chaput de Santonge, D. M., Joyce, C. R., *et al.* (1984). Clinical judgment in rheumatoid arthritis. *Ann. Rheum. Dis.* **43**, 686–94.

Ritchie, D. M., Boyle, J. A., McInnes, J. M., *et al.* (1968). Clinical studies with an articular index for the assessment of joint tenderness in patients with rheumatoid arthritis. *Quart. J. Med.* **147**, 393–406.

Appendix 3. Literature for patients

The Arthritis and Rheumatism Council for Research in Great Britain undertakes the publication of literature informing patients about rheumatic diseases. This takes the form of *booklets* which are designed to be handed out by doctors to patients during the consultation. The booklets discuss rheumatic diseases in general terms, and queries about individual problems will still need to be answered by the patient's own doctor. Limited topics are covered in some shorter *leaflets*.

This literature is available free (apart from postage) to doctors who apply for it from the Arthritis and Rheumatism Council. Applications should be addressed to:

THE GENERAL SECRETARY
ARTHRITIS AND RHEUMATISM COUNCIL
41 EAGLE STREET
LONDON WC1R 4AR

The following booklets and leaflets are available at the time of writing (an up-to-date list will be sent on request):

BOOKLETS

Ankylosing spondylitis.
Are you sitting comfortably? (A guide to choosing easy chairs.)
Backache.
Gout.
Introducing arthritis.
Lupus (SLE).
Osteoarthritis explained.
Pain in the neck.
Rheumatoid arthritis explained.
When your child has arthritis.
Your home and your rheumatism.

LEAFLETS

Polymyalgia rheumatica.
Tennis elbow.
A new hip joint.

FACTSHEETS

In addition, in response to the numerous requests which the Council receives for information directly from patients, it is now preparing a series of short, simple *factsheets* suitable for mailing direct to patients in response to some of the more common enquiries. The first three fact-sheets deal with:

Allergy.
Exercise.
Weather.

ARC magazine

Finally, the authors commend GP's to subscribe to the magazine ARC published by the Council. This includes articles on the work of the Council, research into arthritis and rheumatism, and much information of interest to sufferers from rheumatic diseases. It makes excellent reading matter for the waiting room.

Useful addresses

The Arthritis and Rheumatism Council: 41 Eagle Street, London WC1R 4AR (provide patient's booklets on most forms of arthritis).

British Medical Acupuncture Association: 67–69 Chancery Lane, London WC2 1AF.

British Rheumatism and Arthritis Association: 6 Grosvenor Crescent, London SW1. Tel. 01 235 0902.

The Centre for the Study of Alternative Therapies: 51 Bedford Place, Southampton SO1 2DG.

Disabled Living Foundation: 346 Kensington High Street, London W14 3NS.

General Council and Register of Osteopaths: 1–4 Suffolk Street, London SW1 4HG.

Index

249